10 Essential Foods

A sensible, good-humored approach to vitality, health and well-being.

Lalitha Thomas

HOHM PRESS
PRESCOTT, AZ

10 Essential™, 10 Essential Herbs™ and 10 Essential Foods™
are trademarks of Good Deal Marketing L.L.C.

Design and layout: Visual Perspectives, Phoenix, AZ
Cover design: Kim Johansen

Library of Congress Cataloguing-In- Publication-Data:
Thomas, Lalitha.
  Ten essential foods / Lalitha Thomas.
    p.   cm.
  Includes bibliographical references and index.
  ISBN 0-934252-74-2
  1. Nutrition.   I. Title
RA784.7525   1997
613.2--dc21   95-1005
                                                  CIP

Disclaimer: The theories and formulae in this book are not meant to diagnose, prescribe or to administer in any manner to any physical or psychological ailments. In matters related to health consult a qualified health professional.

Hohm Press
PO Box 2501
Prescott, AZ 86302
1-800-381-2700
http://www.booknotes.com/hohm/

CONTENTS

INTRODUCTION

"How *can* that Lalitha be so bold," you may ask, "to pick ten out of the whole incredible variety of foods in the world and say that they are the *10 Essential* ones!?"

And I will answer, that as far as being bold, it is just one of my more useful eccentricities. As far as being accurate about what is essential, I have learned to recognize these things through more than twenty years of experience and formal apprenticeship to other self-taught Masters in the healing arts, through extensive study in the use of foods and herbs as healing substances (see my first book, *10 Essential Herbs*, Prescott, AZ: Hohm Press, 1992), by lecturing and teaching in this important field, and through consciously applying (since childhood) the highly useful gifts of intuition and flexibility in the use of the healing energies I was born with.

I often just "know things," which has always been quite convenient for me and for those who like to try out my ideas. I have no academic credentials (although I could get good-looking diplomas in the mail, if I was really that interested, and so could you); but I'm making this clear right now, I would never have learned a lot of what is contained in this book if I had depended on traditional, or even not-so-traditional, *academia* to inform me (and I'd bet the same is true for you too).

10 Essential Foods is for those who want positive *action* on the health front that is not only "do-able" and affordable, but easy to keep up on a daily basis wherever in the world we happen to be.

4 GOOD REASONS FOR THE *10 ESSENTIAL FOODS* APPROACH

1. All foods are not equally nutritious. By specifically focusing on 10 of the best foods available today, I encourage you to maximize your health and minimize your need for experimentation and the resulting confusion about your food choices. My herb book, *10 Essential Herbs*, is a huge success partly because it is a simple, straightforward system. I knew the same system would work with foods.

2. In all cultures throughout the world, people are dying unnecessarily from nutrition-related illness such as heart disease, diabetes, cancer and suffering the effects of premature aging. Using these *10 Essential Foods* would greatly lessen those grim statistics.

3. Diets for weight-loss and health enhancement abound. However, many diets are discouraging because they emphasize what not to eat. *10 Essential Foods* emphasizes what you *can* add to your diet and enjoy with gusto! This book is about how to say "Yes" to food!

4. New research is pouring in every day documenting the near-miraculous health-giving properties of phytochemicals and antioxidants in certain foods. I really got inspired to write about what this could mean for our health in practical, "what-should-I-eat-today?" terms.

Of course, many nutritionally extraordinary foods exist in the world, and I certainly enjoy using more than the 10 I emphasize here. What makes these ten the *10 Essential Foods* is that if they are all included regularly in your diet, ideally forming a major influence in all your menu choices, you will experience and appreciate an upscale in health and an ease in maintaining that health.

So, here's the deal! Whether you already know about healthy eating and are able to actually eat well most of the time (no, this does *not* mean the "health hamburgers" from the fast food place!), or whether you are a beginning explorer in this nutritional labyrinth, the *10 Essential Foods* are *the* foods you need to know about.

Children too, can easily become accustomed to enjoying these excellent foods frequently in their diets. Many already do!

WHAT ARE THE 10 ESSENTIAL FOODS?
(And Why I Chose Them)

1. **Almonds**—A complete protein furnishing all the essential amino acids. Since Almonds* can also be sprouted, they have the additional benefits of all the great qualities of sprouts (mentioned in the Sprout chapter). *(Except in sections or chapters specifically devoted to one of the 10 Essential Foods, I will capitalize the names of these 10 throughout the book, to keep drawing your attention to them.)

2. **Broccoli**—Great chlorophyll content and high concentrations of potent disease-preventing phytochemicals. (A few other green vegetables, in the Broccoli family, are equally spectacular, but hey, Broccoli is my favorite and this is my list.)

3. **Brown Rice**—A standout for energy-producing complex carbohydrates, Brown Rice also gets an A+ rating for extraordinary versatility of preparation. You'll find plenty of B vitamins in Brown Rice, along with protein and phytochemicals "up the whazoo" (as a friend of mine says). (Just so we have no misunderstanding, this phrase is how my friend expresses that there are stupendous amounts and varieties of good things in Brown Rices. Throughout the book I sometimes use the plural term "Brown Rices" to keep reminding the reader that there are many types of Brown Rice to choose from.)

4. **Carrots**—A major and easily available source of disease-preventing beta carotene. I wanted a vegetable with a very orange color, because (as I'll discuss later) colors indicate the presence of various phytochemicals, and orange indicates the chemical family of carotenoids, including beta carotene. Besides, I wanted to have all colors present as much as possible and Carrots certainly win a prize in the orange-red category!

5. **Dulse**—One of the rare vegetable sources of vitamin B12, Dulse is especially important for vegetarians. Dulse also furnishes health-crucial trace minerals in abundance and has phytochemicals which offer protection from radioactive pollution.

6. **Figs**—A miracle fruit, Figs have more calcium than milk and wonderful concentrations of other health building major minerals. Unlike many fruits, Figs mix well with most other foods, enhancing digestion through the action of

potent phytochemicals and unique enzymes. Figs are a healthy way to satisfy your "sweet tooth."

7. **Flax Oil**—A special oil containing essential fatty acids, especially the omega 3 group. Essential fatty acids are indispensable to the body's immune functioning and for manufacturing necessary hormones ... along with numerous other jobs.

8. **Grapefruit**—Partly because of vitamin C and bioflavonoid content, I wanted to have a citrus fruit on my list. Among citrus, Grapefruit is of medium acidity, not too sweet, and especially high in vitamin C, bioflavonoids and potent phytochemicals such as quercetin. For the adventurous connoisseur, the seeds and juiceless inner pulp of Grapefruit offer phytochemicals highly valued for their antimicrobial properties.

9. **Spinach**—Superbly green, spinach has a generous chlorophyll content and the health activating qualities that go along with chlorophyll. Important in rejuvenating the health of the blood, Spinach also is remarkable in its folacin content. (In the Spinach chapter you'll find the entire list of what wonders folicin can do for your health!)

10. **Sprouts**—Plant babies! Grow them anywhere; take them anywhere. Sprouts are power houses of nutrients and life force.

In choosing these particular foods I wanted to offer you a broad spectrum of colors because, in addition to the pleasing sight of a vibrant mix of color on your plate, colors indicate variety of phytochemical content and activity. In fact, if you think in terms of eating a wide variety of colors in fruits and vegetables each day, you are well on your way to great nutrition!

I wanted to find ten foods that, altogether, would supply the essential amino acids for complete protein (in Almonds I found a single food that contained them all), all trace minerals and major minerals, essential fatty acids, vitamins, complex carbohydrates, and enzymes, in more than just a token fashion. Antioxidant qualities had to be prominent as well. Besides being nutritionally superior, these *10 Essential Foods* had to be available almost anywhere in the world (perhaps varying in form somewhat), affordable, highly versatile in preparation, flavorful and appealing to a wide range of tastes (kids to grandparents). In other words, I wanted these foods, as a group, to provide a *concentrated* and *significant* plan for achieving optimal health through optimal nutrition.

Used correctly (yes, one *does* need to eat more than a spoonful once a week of "The Ten"; and no, one doesn't use the suggested oil as an excuse to fry one's food!) these *10 Essential Foods* meet and surpass all my criteria.

Throughout the *10 Essential Foods* system, I recommend the simplest, freshest, least contaminated form of the food possible. In most cases, each of the *10 Essentials* is a food that is extraordinary in its fresh, uncooked or unprocessed form, yet still has recognizable benefit if lightly and simply cooked or processed in some way.

For example, in their fresh form, Broccoli, Figs or Spinach offer extraordinary nutrition. In their steamed or baked forms these same foods are still nutritionally significant (yet not as extraordinary as the fresh fruits and vegetables). Brown Rices and other whole grains and dried beans are usually cooked (and therefore processed) since these foods are enhanced through cooking. However, many whole grains and dried beans can be eaten raw as sprouted foods, thereby offering all the attendant benefits of the sprouting process. And for those who desire animal protein, tuna fish packed in water, admittedly processed, still has admirable nutrition potential for our purposes (see Chapter 13, about Meat, Fish, Poultry and Dairy).

10 ESSENTIAL FOODS AND BEYOND! (Or, What Else is in This Book?)

In addition to one in-depth chapter covering each of the *10 Essential Foods*, this book contains:

1. A chapter (Chapter 13) on MEAT, FISH, POULTRY and DAIRY which discusses why these are not included as essential foods in this system, and what positive choices are available for those who still want some of these foods in the diet.

2. A RECOMMENDED BIBLIOGRAPHY of the resources quoted in this book, as well as some excellent cookbooks, guidebooks for dietary change, and suggestions for finding additional in-depth information (written in layperson's terms) on each of the topics covered.

3. APPENDIX A—CLINICS: Here I list specific medical clinics which incorporate nutritional therapies with state-of-the-art allopathic and naturopathic disciplines. Here you can expect to find listings of unconventional approaches right alongside the therapies you may be more familiar with. Although I have not personally visited these clinics, they come recommended from people I highly trust. If I were seriously ill and wanted to seek professional help, these are the places where I would begin my investigations.

4. APPENDIX B—SUPPLIES, RECOMMENDED PRODUCTS, AND HEALTH ACCESSORIES: This is a directory for finding products and supplies I mention throughout the text as well as many items I may not have mentioned, but which are so wonderful that I want my readers to know about them. With this directory you can sit at home and take care of many of your health needs by using the mail order sources I list for just about everything. When you visit your local health food store, this directory will help eliminate the guesswork about which brands to choose, since I offer you my own tried and true recommendations. Here you will also find my suggestions for condiments, oils, minerals, whole grains, sprouting supplies, supplements, Super-Foods and Green-Foods (whole-food concentrates) including Blue Green Algae, Wheat and Barley Grass juice, and phytochemical chewables. (This Super-Food listing, by the way, is the result of years of trial and error on my part in finding potent and easy-to-assimilate Super-Food concentrates that give me the exceptional additional nutrition I may need for extra stressful times, or travel, or to repair the damage from the same.)

 Naysayers and friends alike often warn me that I shouldn't be so free with my opinions, nor so specific in naming my favorite types and sources of the goodies described in *10 Essential Foods*. Yet, here I am, in Appendix B, doing it anyway, and proud of it!

5. APPENDIX C—10 ESSENTIAL SNACKS: Everyone will appreciate finding an entire appendix devoted to snacks! This appendix is one that you will love so much you may find yourself recommending my book to every friend, relative, or child-care center you know! If the truth be known, this is one of my favorite parts of the whole book, and was exquisitely fun to make up. The snacks I describe here are *anything but* those fat-producing, addiction-building,

depression-contributing and health-degenerating non-foods that the word "snacks" usually brings to mind. In fact, the 10 Essential Snacks can be an important part of daily nutrition.

6. SURVIVAL CHOICE LISTINGS: We all go through times when we need the convenience of "fast" food, prepackaged meals, or find ourselves with limited food choices, especially when traveling or eating out. For these situations, I include a Survival Choice list at the end of each chapter. The afore-mentioned "survival" situations may call for some sort of compromise to the ideal, and the Survival Choice is just that—the best compromise I can think of to handle an other-wise challenging situation.

If you find *10 Essential Foods* to be as helpful as I designed it to be, you may be interested in using its companion vol-ume, *10 Essential Herbs* (Prescott, AZ: Hohm Press, 1992). In *10 Essential Herbs* I have outlined a simple and immediately usable system for putting your health back to rights on those occasions when you or your family need specific help. As you discover the medicinal uses for these ten common herbs (peppermint, garlic, ginger, etc.) you may well find that you never need anything else for average daily health maintenance. Colds, flu, digestive upsets, muscle pain, stuffy nose, nausea, enhancing immunity, you name it ... this book has an effective herbal treatment for it. And just think, the money you save on doctor bills you can put towards enhancing your *10 Essential Foods* budget!

HOW TO START ... SLOWLY AND SANELY

As they begin to make desired changes in their diets and food habits, many people ask me if they have to start eating all ten of the *10 Essential Foods* every day? To which I reply: Of course not! I advocate a sane, gentle approach to change. The one-step-at-a-time approach. Start small. Start slowly. And above all, don't worry. All of the ten foods don't have to be in your digestive system at the same time, or even on the same day, in order to provide the optimal availability of functional components for superb health. If your overall dietary intake, let's say over a week's time, is well endowed with the *10 Essential Foods*, you will be providing a huge variety of raw materials which your body can utilize according to its own priorities.

If the *10 Essential Foods* suggestions are new to you, I recommend that you pick the friendliest looking food on the list and start with a once-a-week try (once-a-day if you are feeling particularly bold). In this way you can painlessly sneak up on yourself with dietary additions of the *10 Essential Foods* in a mood of fun-loving investigation. This is the same basic advice I gave to my friend Jane, whose story follows.

TASOLE: [The word is "TASOLE" (pronounced tassel). It stands for **T**rue **A**ctual **S**tories **O**f **L**alitha's **E**xperiences. Each chapter contains one or more such stories about food adventures which will assist the reader in easily remembering the basic concepts upon which this book is based.]

Jane was a high profile woman with a high responsibility job that kept her going at top speed for ten hours a day. One day I received a "distress" call from her.

"Lalitha, my health seems to be crumbling more every day!" Jane blurted out frantically. "I eat breakfast with my morning coffee but by 10 A.M. the sugar craving starts and I can't resist the candy bar machine. After lunch I'm running out of energy again about 2 P.M., and again I rush to the snack machine. I'm gaining weight like crazy and ..."

"Wait, wait a minute," I interrupted her. "Is this the Jane who just last week was telling me that junk food snacks agreed with her very well because she simply "burned it all off" with all the work she had to do in a day?"

"Well, ... er," Jane mumbled, "I guess I *am* noticing that the energy bursts from my snacks are short-lived. But how else can I get through my day?"

"First tell me this," I asked. "What kind of breakfast are you having with your coffee and what are you calling lunch these days?"

"Breakfast is a sweet roll and a cup of coffee. Lunch is usually pasta, and maybe a soda, or sometimes a deli sandwich," Jane described.

At my end of the telephone I rolled my eyes in mock amazement. I was not terribly surprised that Jane wasn't getting enough nutrition in her first two meals of the day. At this point I hesitated to ask her about her dinner habits.

"I think you would get more stable energy output from your basic meals if you could make a couple of additions, or changes," I said. "I'm not crazy enough to try and mess around with all your dietary habits, since I know you're sensitive about that. But, could you just keep in the back of your mind that you might do better, stamina-wise, with protein foods such as tuna, or Almonds, along with vegetables at breakfast and/or lunch."

Jane let out an exasperated sigh as she replied, "But I'm always in such a rush and besides, who ever heard of eating vegetables, besides fried potatoes that is, for breakfast?"

"Just keep it in mind," I repeated. "Listen, in case you get inspired, I'll tell you my list of *10 Essential Foods* and maybe there will come a day when you can try one or two along with your usual meals." I gave her the list and hung up.

I didn't hear from Jane for about three weeks, so I assumed she was continuing on as usual. Then, seemingly out of the blue, I got another call.

"Lalitha, that list is great!" she sounded like she was trying to sell me something.

For my part, I couldn't remember which list she was referring to until she continued, "You know, your '10 favorite foods' list. I tried it!"

"Why did you do that?! I mean, what happened?" I asked, genuinely surprised and still a little confused.

"One weekend I felt so worn out that I stayed home for a change. That's when I took time to look at your list," Jane admitted. "I added steamed Broccoli, raw Almonds and fresh Carrots to my meals on Saturday. On Sunday I really got inspired and had a piece of broiled fish and even put some Sprouts on my salad. You would have been proud of that salad. It was much better than the pile of iceberg lettuce I usually have. Simply adding those foods to my diet over the weekend made a noticeable difference in how I felt."

"What happened when you got back to work on Monday?" I asked, wondering if maybe it was just the rest during the weekend that had done it.

"I tried a new restaurant for one thing," Jane laughed. I found one near my office that had a great salad bar and broiled fish. Several people I work with regularly eat there. Anyway, during the week I tried your list idea by adding some dried Figs to my diet, and wow, what a difference that made! I don't think I'll ever go back to the snacks from the candy machine. Two or three Figs seemed to keep me from crashing at energy lows during the day, and I still felt good an hour or so after when I usually would be having that sugar-low feeling again."

I heartily agreed. The Fig idea had saved me on many a high-stress occasion when I couldn't stop to eat a meal.

"I've got to go now," Jane finished, "I'm off to another staff meeting. But I wanted to tell you I'm passing a copy of your list on to my mom!"

Phytochemicals, vitamins, minerals, amino acids, enzymes— a few of the *functional components* which account for the optimal nutritional content of certain foods—are some of the reasons why Jane and others receive such rewards from expanding their food choices to include more of the *10 Essential Foods* in their daily diet.

In proceeding slowly with dietary changes, as Jane did, you give your body time to adjust to a healing and changing body chemistry. For example, for some people, eating healthier foods gives the body a signal that it can proceed with long-overdue repair work. When the body's attention is taken up with simply surviving the ravages of poor food choices, it doesn't have the time or energy to do anything but the most minimal repair work.

When done too quickly, this rebuilding process can be uncomfortable, especially if one is cutting down on refined sugars, meats or milk products. With slow steady changes, however, most discomfort is avoided and people are more likely to notice how great they are feeling!

For more specific help in making changes, or for improving a diet that is already headed in a healthy direction, a fine resource is the book *Intuitive Eating* by Dr. Humbart "Smokey" Santillo, N.D. (Prescott, AZ: Hohm Press, 1993). Every food-lover and new food-explorer can profit from this book. Using one or more of the book's concise charts, you can discover exactly where you are starting from regarding your present diet. Next, Dr. Santillo will guide you step-by-step along the path of improvement while providing examples of meals plans for each stage. His comprehensive research and instruction will leave you with no doubt about the "whys and wherefores" for every change. Such an education will make you quite skilled at navigating life with vitality-enhancing dietary habits. Over time, these habits do indeed become "intuitive," as the title suggests, and therefore highly portable and usable at any stage of life and in every circumstance.

The good news of the *10 Essential Foods* system is that you can start making a difference in your health today! You don't have to stop to study nutritional science, unless you want to. The healing, life-saving, health-transforming, complex functional components in the *10 Essential Foods* will go to work for you regardless of how much you know about them. Adding one or two of these food to your daily diet is the safe and sure place to start.

"WHAT IF I WANT MORE VARIETY or DISLIKE ONE OF THE 10 ESSENTIALS?"

Occasionally someone says to me that they strongly dislike one of the *10 Essential Foods*, or would like further variety. For instance, I have a friend who claims that eating Almonds makes her throat itch. A few people have found my suggestion of including Dulse (a type of seaweed, or "sea vegetable," as I prefer) a bit unusual and have therefore left it untried. My reply is always, "No problem." At the end of each chapter I include a section called: **HEALTHY ADDITIONS AND TRAVELERS TIPS,** which can be used to make this approach more individualized, or intelligently expanded. In this section, a Healthy Addition is one which is generally quite close in outstanding traits to the food the chapter is named for. If you cannot eat, just don't want to eat, or would like additional variety to the "ideal" food described in each chapter, you will generally find a Healthy Addition that suits you, while serving a similar purpose. For example, in the case of the Almonds and the itching throat, my friend found that she loved eating ground sesame seeds sprinkled onto her vegetables, instead. For the person somewhat timid about trying Dulse at first, there is raw or steamed red Swiss chard, or kale (not identical but excellent alternatives, or Healthy Additions). For those, like myself, who delight in the limitless variety this system entails, the HEALTHY ADDITIONS AND TRAVELERS TIPS point the direction for endless culinary extravaganzas.

I can almost guarantee that you will not feel deprived or bored in eating the *10 Essential Foods*. (Although if you are bored for reasons other than food, I can't do too much about it, except to say that many psychological conditions seem to mysteriously disappear when the body starts getting its full complement of essential nutrients.)

First of all, eating as much as you want, as often as you want (and I really think you should go for it), of the *10 Essential Foods*, their Healthy Additions, the Super-Foods (special concentrated foods, see Appendix B), and the 10 Essential Snacks would add up to nearly limitless combinations and varieties. No boredom in sight! In fact, in choosing the foods for this book I kept in mind that I wanted foods which, in general, could be eaten almost without limit. (Well, as much as a sane person would want, anyway. My friend Bill ate only piles of Broccoli everyday for a week or so, and this is not what I am talking about.) When you eat as much as you want, as often as you want, of foods that not only make you feel wonderful but discourage weight gain, there's not much room left for feeling deprived. A feeling of abundance more closely describes what you can expect with this plan. (I expand on this idea at the beginning of chapter 2.)

This book is about saying "YES" to food! Saying "YES" to putting vitality *into* the body (in the form of food), and to receiving vitality (that means, *LIFE*) back.

1

A BIT OF NUTRITIONAL BACKGROUND

THE SHORT COURSE

This chapter will cover some of the basics of food and nutrition, and will hopefully get you so inspired and excited about these *10 Essential Foods* ideas that you may find yourself telling everyone you know about them. Watch out for the hazard of making a pest of yourself, however. If your best friend, who is eating a candy bar and guzzling a soft drink, starts to glare (or snarl) at you while you expound on the virtues of phytochemicals, this is your first clue to "get a grip on yourself" and try turning down your enthusiasm control for the time being.

On the other hand, if you are the type for whom this sort of nutritional information is a bit overwhelming, no harm is done if you skip this chapter altogether. Perhaps you will want to come back to it later. No pressure. Don't worry.

UP THE PYRAMID

Here and there throughout this book I refer to the USDA (United States Department of Agriculture) "Food Guide Pyramid" which was put together by their Human Nutrition Information Service. (See Figure 1.1)

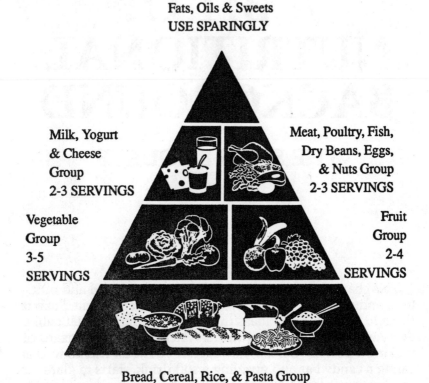

Fats, Oils & Sweets
USE SPARINGLY

Milk, Yogurt
& Cheese
Group
2-3 SERVINGS

Meat, Poultry, Fish,
Dry Beans, Eggs,
& Nuts Group
2-3 SERVINGS

Vegetable
Group
3-5
SERVINGS

Fruit
Group
2-4
SERVINGS

Bread, Cereal, Rice, & Pasta Group
6-11 SERVINGS

figure 1.1 Food Guide Pyramid. Re-drawn form USDA Publication
No. HG-252. Hyattsville, MD: USDA, 1992

The U.S. Surgeon General estimates that 66% of all deaths in the United States are diet related! The Food Guide Pyramid is the beginning of a nation-wide project to re-educate Americans about what a healthy diet is supposed to be, replacing the old "4 Food Groups" system. You remember that don't you? The 4 Food Groups: vegetables, fruits, grains, and the animal-based proteins of meats, eggs, and dairy products. You probably also remember the great emphasis placed on eating hefty amounts of this fourth (or protein) group. Everywhere we looked advertisements told us to drink several glasses of milk every day, and to eat meat or eggs in some form with practically every meal! Fats, oils and sweets were frequently and casually used in those "good ol' days." In fact, fats and sweets were almost an unofficial food group in themselves for many households.

With the health of Americans steadily declining and degenerative diseases on an epidemic rise, more people are taking a second look at this all-American diet. Research is now confirming that diet is at the core of a lot of our health problems, with the high intake of animal-based foods, often high in fat, as the leading "killers." The outrageous consumption of processed sugars is also a leading contender.

It took a long time for us, the general public, to start taking seriously the information pouring in from research centers here and abroad which was telling us loud and clear that our dietary choices (particularly the high intake of fats, concentrated animal proteins, and processed sugars) were poisoning us! Finally, however, the evidence became so overwhelming that U.S. government agencies began to officially warn of the health hazards of our typical dietary choices. Many of the most common chronic degenerative diseases such as heart disease, obesity and arthritis are now clearly linked to poor nutrition.

At the same time as they were confirming this unpleasant news, these government agencies began to develop a many-faceted plan for re-education in these matters of diet and health, for both adults and children. This is where the new Food Pyramid comes into play. This model graphically portrays what are now 5 Major Food Groups, and, perhaps more importantly, clearly shows a healthier scheme for figuring out the proportions of intake necessary from each group. For instance, you can see on the chart the major role that grains, fruits, and vegetables should play in the daily diet and the relatively small role the meat/dairy group plays. Fats, oils and sweets comprise a tiny spot at the top with a note to "Use

Sparingly." In other words, it is not suggested that we need to eat from this group every day!

Overall, I think this Food Pyramid is a giant step ahead in our government's official output regarding our health. At the same time, I know that many compromises had to be made among the politicians, dairy producers, beef farmers, etc. to get the information out at all. (I mean, all those food producers don't want their food group to be lessened, or to have any health hazard associated with it. After all, these producers have spent millions of dollars training us to eat more milk, eggs and meat.) Consumers need to know that the Food Pyramid is much better advice than we previously had, but is still a compromised story.

In spite of my criticisms, I heartily support the use of the principles embodied in the Food Guide Pyramid. Furthermore, with the help of the more specific, detailed and eye-opening information for super-charged health that you will find here in *10 Essential Foods*, you will be able to refine your "Pyramid choices" several degrees more than the government suggests, without compromising the generalized principles embodied in the Pyramid. (For your own copy of several different government Home and Garden publications explaining these new dietary guidelines, write to: USDA, Human Nutrition Information Service, 6505 Belcrest Road, Hyattsville, MD 20782. Or, inquire about this information through your own local USDA county extension office.)

WHY ARE FRESH FOODS THE BEST?

Knowing the basic foods and the general proportions we should eat, according to the Food Pyramid, is a good first step in our nutritional education. Next, and vitally important, we need to address the quality of those foods. In a nutshell, the more available "functional components" a food contains, the higher its overall quality and usability by the body.

"Functional component" is the name applied to any part of a food which contributes to bodily processes—digestive processes, eliminative processes, and specific chemical processes resulting in production of energy, support of the immune system, hormone production, etc. Functional components may or may not (like non-nutritive fiber, for instance) have a specific nutritive value. You have probably heard of phytochemicals, antioxidants, vitamins, minerals, fibers, enzymes, protein, essential fatty acids, etc. These are names for general groups of functional components, each of which has from a few to thousands of individual components: vitamin A, beta carotene, calcium, etc.

Fresh (uncooked) foods, especially those allowed to grow to their peak of maturity before harvest, contain the highest concentrations and widest variety of functional components, and are the health-builders and health-preservers of the body.

The way foods are grown, harvested, transported, stored, prepared, or commercially processed all influence the quality and quantity of the functional components. Since most of these circumstances are not in the control of the consumer, the smart shopper will take a pro-active role as soon as possible—by buying the freshest available foods, and avoiding unnecessary processing, cooking and additives which can detract further from the nutritional quality of the food. For instance, cooking will not affect most minerals, but vitamin C is significantly destroyed with only a little heat. Another example: while proper fats and oils are essential to a healthy diet, the processing ("refining") of those oils turns them into a "liver-stressing nightmare" before we even get them unpackaged; the cooking of the fats after we get them home compounds the horror. Learning about *what* fresh food is, *how* to find it, and *how* to keep it that way is what this book is all about.

In the chapters that follow I go into more detail on the selection, preparation and consumption of foods. Familiarity with these important details will allow you to reap an optimal harvest of functional components for the encouragement of your optimal health.

THE PHYTOCHEMICAL REVOLUTION

Recently, a seemingly new category of functional components called *phytochemicals* (*phyto* comes from the Greek word for plant) has been taking the nutritional world by storm; showing up in new health products and written about in hundreds of health and diet-related articles in the popular news media.

However, the idea of phytochemicals is only seemingly new. Enlightened physicians, at least as far back as Hippocrates (Greek physician, circa 460-370 BC), have used the healing and protective powers (which included phytochemical activity) in whole foods. Hippocrates is famous for his statement: "Let your food be your medicine and your medicine be your food."

So, what's the big deal about phytochemicals all of a sudden?

The "big deal" is that our so-called modern science is isolating, researching, tracking the activity of, and naming these hundreds of substances faster than they can update their lists.

While the knowledge of phytochemicals and their beneficial results for health may not be new, the public's interest in knowing about them is. Information on this flush of new research is pouring forth from such prestigious research foundations as the Harvard Medical School, the University of Illinois Functional Foods For Health (FFH) program, Johns Hopkins Medical Institution, the Cancer Research Institute, and our own United States Department of Agriculture.

In fact, if you are on-line with the Internet you can access one of the most outstanding phytochemical databases in the world, for free. This list was compiled over many years by James Duke, Ph.D., folk-hero *extraordinaire* and a world-renowned phytochemical researcher, author, and lecturer. (His exploits in and out of rain forests have even made him the subject of an epic poem.) Dr. Duke is now retired from his thirty or more years at the USDA, where he and his associates were funded to do the extensive laboratory and field research for this database. When I was lucky enough to get him on the telephone to ask him some phytochemical questions, he told me that he had "left his ghost" available on the Internet, free to anyone who cared to look at it, and that it was still continually updated by his colleagues! Duke emphasized that his primary interest, now that he was "retired," was to continue his work in rain forests, studying rain forest phytochemicals and their possible uses for medicine. His database is generated out of the Phytochemeco Database at the National Germplasm Resources Laboratory USDA, Agricultural Research Service. It is called "Phytochemical and Ethnobotanical Databases." The internet address is: http://www.ars-grin.gov/~ngrlsb/

Use this database to answer any questions about any plant substance you can think of—be it food, herbal medicine, whatever. Dr. Duke's help to me, however brief, certainly added to the fascinating facts I have compiled in this book.

Long before functional components became a popular subject for current research, many contemporary health professionals had used these components of fruits, vegetables, herbs, oils, etc. extensively, with profound results in human health. For example, seven-time Nobel Award nominated physician, biochemist and nutritionist Dr. Johanna Budwig, M.D., Ph.D., has received worldwide acclaim for her work with essential fatty acids and their applications in the treatment of cancer and other diseases. A major source of these essential fatty acids in her work is from specially processed flaxseed oil. (For in-depth information, in layperson's terms, on Dr. Budwig's disease fighting program, see: *Flax Oil as a True Aid Against Arthritis, Heart Infarction, Cancer and other Diseases*. Vancouver, B.C. Canada: Apple Publishing, 1992. Available through Barlean's Oils 1-800-445-3529.)

The phytochemicals found in plants (fruits and vegetables) are "bio-active" in profound ways, different from the mysterious, remarkable and more commonly researched actions of vitamins, minerals, enzymes, etc. Unlike nutrients which nourish the whole body, phytochemicals support *specific* functions. For example, some phytochemicals enhance the immune system in dramatic ways. Others provide the micro-nutrients designed to support the body's natural production of hormones.

Crucial to good health in both plants and humans, phytochemicals are only present in micro-amounts. (In case you are thinking that "micro-amounts" sounds like something that you can probably do without, with no problem, just pinch that little thought out of your brain right now!) Nutrition is deficient without phytochemicals, period! (*Sigh, ugh, oh well ...* Someone will probably feel compelled to write to me about that statement. I know there are still some researchers who maintain that phytochemicals technically have nothing to do with nutrition, because they are not yet known to be necessary for health, as are the more commonly known nutrients such as vitamins, minerals, fatty acids, etc. Whoever these researchers are, they'll have to catch up with us later.) In other words, phytochemicals are present in excruciatingly tiny amounts in plants and these same small amounts in the diets of humans can contribute to outstandingly good health! Happily, therefore, you won't have to eat a pound of carrots a day, for instance, in order to get a health-beneficial dose of the beta carotene which carrots can provide. For a healthy person, one medium-size Carrot could be enough to fulfill one day's maintenance needs for beta carotene.

Phytochemicals are largely responsible for a plant's color. Simply by eating five or more different colors of fruits and/or vegetables each day, you will be getting the benefit of five different phytochemicals (who cares what their names are!). Phytochemicals are also largely responsible for a plant's odor, flavor, and the healing capacity of many medicinal herbs, since they are the main self-defense system in plants. So, eating phytochemical-rich plants you reap the same highly potent, self-defense activity for your cells that the plants enjoy. (Serious protection here!)

Although much is still unknown about how all the functional components work together, overwhelming evidence exists for the ability of phytochemicals (whether they have yet been "discovered" and named or not) to protect us from developing diseases such as cancer, heart disease, macular degeneration, diabetes and others. For instance, current research and articles about phytochemicals and disease can be found in: *Harvard Health News Letter*, April 1995, "Cancer Fighting Foods," 9-12; *Dynamic Chiropractic*, April 24, 1995, "Phytochemical Review"; *Journal of American Medical Association* (JAMA), April 12, 1995, "Protective Effects of Fruits and Vegetables on Development of Stroke in Men"; *JAMA*, November 9, 1994, "Dietary Carotenoids, Vitamins A, C, and E, and Advanced Age-Related Macular Degeneration"; *JAMA*, November 9, 1994, "Serum Carotenoids and Coronary Heart Disease"; *McCall's*, December 1994, "The Healing Power of Fruits and Vegetables," 46-47; *Newsweek*, April 1994, "Beyond Vitamins," 45-49, to cite only a few sources.

When the phytochemicals, vitamins, minerals and all the other functional components of optimal nutrition are available to do their synergistic magic in us, the rejuvenating effects are dramatic—bordering on flamboyant, I would say! In each of the food chapters that follow, I will point out the major functional components of that food, including phytochemicals and antioxidants, and describe what these substances are so far known to protect against. I will also list the major vitamins and minerals contained in each of the *10 Essential Foods*.

ANTIOXIDANTS—THEY CAPTURE FREE RADICALS!

Antioxidants too are getting much publicity these days, as their importance becomes undeniably obvious. Antioxidants are usually mentioned in the same breath as "free radicals" and "free-radical scavengers," because antioxidants *are* free-radical scavengers—i.e., they scavenge or "capture" free radicals.

The business of free-radical scavengers and free radicals takes place on the subcellular level. A free radical is an oxygen molecule with an unpaired electron inside it which causes that particular oxygen molecule to behave in a violent fashion, bashing around amongst other molecules, trying to find another oxygen molecule to join up with to create a stable situation... in the electron department, that is. Scientists made up the name "free radicals" for these unstable oxygen molecules. So there you have it.

Some free-radical activity is healthy and natural to bodily processes and other free-radical activity is not. For our purposes we are mainly concerned with the unhealthy type of free-radical activity; so from now on, when I talk about free radicals, understand I'm talking about the free-radical "bad guys." The violent activity of these free radicals creates all sorts of oxidizing damage to our cells, hampering cellular processes and disintegrating cellular tissues, thus causing the signs of deterioration we call aging and/or illness. We need free-radical scavengers to round up these *crazies* (the unwanted free radicals) and neutralize them. This is where antioxidants come into play. In my mind, anti-oxidant = against oxygen damage, or against free-radical damage—get it?

Although the human body produces antioxidants, this supply is often inadequate given the large number of circumstances which escalate free-radical activity. To remedy this, we can take antioxidant supplements or eat foods high in antioxidant substances (more about this later). Yet, even with the ready availability of antioxidants, both internally and externally, we still need education in how to preserve our health. It's a free-radical jungle out there. Kenneth H. Cooper M.D., well-known health investigator and author of several books, writes in his book *Antioxidant Revolution* (Nashville, TN: Thomas Nelson Publishers, 1994, pp.10-11):

> Unfortunately, the normal internal and external protective systems often are not adequate. The problem is that too many free radicals may be generated by such factors as air pollution, cigarette smoke, ultraviolet light produced by the sun, pesticides and other contaminants in your food—even too much exercise. [*And, Lalitha adds, over-cooked and processed foods, cooked oils, especially fried oils and junk foods of all types, certainly contribute directly and indirectly to this sorry state of affairs.*] It seems that everywhere we turn, substances and situations threaten to flood our bodies with free radicals.
>
> When your body becomes overwhelmed by extra free radicals, those unstable oxygen molecules are transformed from your allies into molecular predators. They begin to run wild,

successfully attacking healthy as well as unhealthy parts of the body. Heart disease, various cancers, and many other diseases are frequently the result.

This is where using the *10 Essential Foods* comes in. All ten are loaded with top-notch antioxidants, and eating lots of them and their Healthy Additions will greatly increase your antioxidant intake and give you a huge free-radical-scavenging capacity!

In addition to the efficient antioxidants the body itself produces, antioxidants available from our foods and supplements include all sorts of phytochemicals, vitamins, minerals, enzymes and co-enzymes such as beta carotene, vitamin C, vitamin E, selenium, co-enzyme Q10, bioflavonoids, and zinc, to name a few.

Antioxidant Content: How To Recognize It and How To Keep It!

The following lists will assist you in choosing foods with the highest antioxidant content, and preparing that food so that the antioxidant content is preserved as much as possible.

Choosing Great Food:

1. Go for color. Eat a large variety of vibrant colors and right away you can know that you are expanding your phytochemical/antioxidant intake. Examples of good color choices are: red onions over white onions; red grapes over the green or white ones; dark green leafy vegetables; like Spinach, Sprouts, parsley, and leaf lettuces over the watery-green stuff such as iceberg lettuce and pink Grapefruit over the lighter varieties
2. Use fresh and frozen fruits and vegetables, which have higher nutrient and antioxidant activity than canned, processed, sweetened or cooked selections. Choose fresh unrefined oils such as Flax oil or extra virgin olive oil over the commonly available vegetable oil mixtures from the grocery store.
3. Choose fresh raw nuts and seeds over the roasted and salted ones.
4. Choose raw or lightly cooked vegetables over heavily cooked, canned, or processed ones.

Preserving Top Antioxidant Content in Foods:

In *The Antioxidant Revolution*, Dr. Cooper tells us exactly how to preserve as many of the vital antioxidants (and therefore most other vital functional components) as possible by keeping the following points in mind in food preparation. His suggestions coincide perfectly (no surprise) with other food experts such as Humbart Santillo, author of *Intuitive Eating* (Prescott, AZ: Hohm Press, 1984), Jean Carper (*Food Your Miracle Medicine*. NY: Harper Collins, 1993), and Carol Nostrand (*Junk Food to Real Food*. New Canaan, CT: Keats Publishers, 1994). I'll paraphrase, summarize and ad-lib:

1. Avoid wilted produce and *do not buy* pre-cut produce.
2. Don't trim off or discard the highly useful and edible skins, outer leaves, etc. Eat them as part of the dish you are preparing. Exceptions to this are non-organic produce which cannot be cleaned of offending chemical coatings, such as the skins of waxed apples and cucumbers. I make case-by-case judgments on this "to trim-or-not-to-trim question" with non-organic produce depending on how effective I think my cleaning methods have been and how offending some of the coatings are. Even so, most waxed coatings get trimmed off.
3. Don't cook foods with the "swimming in water" methods. Use as little water as needed, or use a steamer basket which holds foods up out of the water, thereby keeping the nutrition in the food instead of in the cooking water, which is often thrown away. Add any leftover cooking water back to the food whenever possible. Antioxidants will be present in it!
4. Avoid excessive heat in cooking. Long boiling, or other extended cooking, or exposing foods to flame or smoke can damage antioxidants. DO NOT FRY FOODS.
5. Use syrups or liquids that result from thawing frozen foods.
6. Do not refrigerate once-cooked foods for more than a day, and always store them in air-tight containers.
7. Try not to reheat once-cooked fruit or vegetable dishes.
8. Avoid keeping foods warm for more than thirty minutes before you serve them, as antioxidants are being lost increasingly with this passage of time.
9. Do not hold fresh produce in your refrigerator for more than a few days, and certainly not longer than a week. Buying frozen fruits and vegetables is a better choice if you think you won't consume the fresh produce within a few days of purchase.

For the full scoop about antioxidants refer to Dr. Kenneth Cooper's *Antioxidant Revolution* (Nashville, TN: Thomas Nelson Publishers, 1994), and Humbart Santillo's *Intuitive Eating* (Prescott, AZ: Hohm Press, 1993).

THE IMMUNE SYSTEM

With all this valuable information about phytochemicals, antioxidants and other functional components, I want to give you a firmer, core-level understanding for why all of this is important—namely, the health of your immune system.

When the immune system is functioning optimally, health traumas of all sorts can be prevented or handled quite efficiently by the body. Whether the traumas are from stress, emotions, "germs," junk food, a cranky boss, or whatever, the body has the potential to produce substances that can neutralize, transform, or just plain dismantle the resultant health-deteriorating chemistry. Even regarding serious illness that seems just to "pop up out of the blue," I still hold that an effective immune system might have prevented such an illness. It takes time, sometimes a long time, for many of those seemingly "just popped up" conditions to develop; and during that time the disease process could have been stopped by a hardy immune system.

Diabetes, arthritis, cancer, heart disease—yes, these are all diet related. Often we are not getting, or absorbing, the functional components from our foods that could actually build an immunity which would prevent the ravages of even these "biggies." On the other hand, if we were getting all these wonderful phytochemicals, antioxidants, vitamins, etc., in our diet, our immune system wouldn't have to work so hard fixing things up in the first place.

I don't believe that everyone needs to become a vegetarian to have the type of immunity I am describing, although some fascinating research does support the vegetarian cause. In Jean Carper's book *Food Your Miracle Medicine* (NY: Harper Collins, 1993), she reports on research at the German Cancer Research Center in Heidelberg which compared the blood of male vegetarians with that of meat-eaters. The white blood cells of the vegetarians were twice as deadly against tumor cells as those of the meat-eaters. Besides the white blood cell activity, these researchers analyzed the blood for the amount of the powerful antioxidant, carotene, which comes from vegetables. The vegetarians, of course, had much higher levels of carotenes in their blood, and because of the disease-preventing qualities of carotenes (see chapter 5), it was surmised that this contributed to the increased effectiveness of the white blood cells in the vegetarians. In other words, it took half as many of the "vegetarian white blood cells" to do the same work as the "non-vegetarian white blood cells." What this means to me is that non-vegetarians simply need to eat lots more vegetables and perhaps less animal-based food. (Throughout my book, you will find that I quote the extraordinary results of Jean Carper's investigations into health research from all over the world. No other book, in my opinion, offers the sheer scope of information gathered into one place. For me it was a beneficial coincidence when I got to sit next to her at a health trade show where we were each signing copies of our respective books. This is where I first became aware of her work.)

The 1996 update of the *Dietary Guidelines for Americans* more clearly endorses the healthful advantage of a vegetarian diet and also urges us to exercise more and avoid weight gain as we grow older. Further, these guidelines suggest lowering alcohol intake, limiting salt/sodium intake, and avoiding trans-fatty acids in partially hydrogenated and hydrogenated oils (see more about this in chapter 9: Flax Oil).

None of these suggestions came as any surprise to us long-time whole-foods aficionados. What is wonderful news to health advocates, concerned parents and researchers alike is that this more enlightened viewpoint is being taught to the children in our schools. These guidelines indicate that a small few, but significant, steps have been taken in overcoming the politics, i.e., the manipulative influences, of certain big business interests.

People with extraordinary immunity will generally not develop illness even if they are sneezed on or coughed on by others who are ill with a serious infection. This is the kind of immunity potential we all possess, but which many of us cancel out every time we sit down to a meal of processed, de-vitalized, trans-fat-saturated, functional-component-deficient foods. And, extraordinary immunity may be our only defense against the virulent new strains of diseases which are sweeping the world—diseases which are increasingly resistant to treatments of any sort. In his 1996 *Director-General's Message for The World Health Report*, Hiroshi Nakajima, M.D. Ph.D., of the World Health Organization (WHO) made this quite clear when he forcefully announced that we:

... stand on the brink of a global crisis in infectious diseases. No country is safe. No country can any longer afford to ignore their threat ... Infectious diseases are attacking us on multiple fronts. Together they represent the world's leading cause of premature death. [Antibiotics] ... are becoming less and less effective as resistance to them spreads. Meanwhile evidence gathers on the role of viruses, bacteria and parasites in the genesis of deadly cancers of the stomach, cervix and liver.

Even though some readers may protest that I am giving them nightmares with this kind of information, my main point is that: within our bodies there is the potential for extraordinary immunity to most of these "attackers." Almost anyone can improve this immunity. The *10 Essential Foods*, along with their Healthy Additions, can play an important role in this.

SUPPLEMENTS VS. THE REAL THING

Nutritional supplements of all types are gaining enthusiastic advocates every day. Deficiencies in the foods available to us, poor diets in general, and the nutrient-devouring stress of our lifestyle are a few of the good reasons. However, anyone who has tried to figure out which supplements to take for which condition knows that there can be no end to the confusion. To say nothing of the potentially huge cost of being well-supplemented! Just when we think we have found the best, newest, most well-researched, and most potent forms of the XYZ nutrients available (the ones that will surely hold us together and protect our health in the years to come), one look at the resultant pile of pills we will be forced to swallow each day (and sometimes several times a day) may bring on a bout of nausea. That's when many of us decide to re-think our strategy. After all, we need to leave some room for "real food" don't we?

Be wary and wise. All the functional components I mention throughout this book are available as supplement tablets at health stores. And, supplement tablets simply cannot do the same job that whole foods can do (so don't even *dream* such a fallacy). The components I mention are all contained *within whole foods*, which means they are working together in synergistic balance with a myriad of other known and unknown components within those foods. Having said that, I want to make it clear that I am not at all against taking supplements. I have used them in moderation (and yes, I must admit, sometimes in excess) with huge benefit (I wouldn't ever want to be without my Klamath Blue-Green Algae tablets!).

For those who go overboard in the supplement department, however, I can't stop myself from repeating the following story told by Dr. Joel Wallach D.V.M., N.D. This story indicates why a consumer of supplements must be educated. For example, we need to know the sources of our supplements (whether the calcium we are taking is from rocks or plants, etc.). We need to know what "binders" or excipients (inert substances which give the supplement its bulk or desired consistency) are present.

One day, Dr. Wallach talked to a man who ran a portable chemical toilet business. (I'll call the man John.) Somehow the subject turned to vitamins.

John told Dr. Wallach that vitamins couldn't be doing people any good because they rarely dissolved. When Dr. Wallach asked him how he knew this, John took him out into the yard where the cleaning of the portable toilets took place. There, Wallach was amazed to see what he called "a mountain of vitamin pills" which had been caught on a quarter-inch screen used inside each toilet for catching any non-dissolvable items, like children's toys, flashlights, coins, etc. John pointed out that he could still read imprints on some of these vitamin tablets, many of which were the products of well-known drug companies!

Personally, I prefer "whole-food supplements," or "Super-Foods" as they are sometimes called, over the common vitamin or mineral supplements. (Some of my long-standing favorites are listed under Super-Foods in Appendix B.) These Super-Foods have all their "parts," so to speak, which usually enables them to be more easily assimilated and used in the body.

In addition to a whole-food supplement, I most often take additional magnesium with some calcium (in tablet form), and liquid ionic trace minerals. During the fall to winter seasonal change, or for high stress travel, I will commonly use a potent antioxidant. For me, simple is better; I quickly wilt when faced with a pile of pills to swallow.

Years ago I learned an easy "dissolve test" which I try on all my new supplements. I soak a few tablets in a cup of water to which I add about 1 teaspoon of vinegar to simulate the digestive juices in the human stomach. (In many people the digestive juices seem no more efficient than plain water, so adding the vinegar to my dissolve test is giving everybody the benefit of the doubt, i.e., assuming that we all have a little acid in our stomachs). If a tablet shows little or extremely slow evidence of breaking down in my home-grown test, this doesn't bode well for its internal absorption. I definitely think twice about using such a supplement.

Ill persons may take supplements to help them feel better, but it is easy for them to fall into over-doing it. Many health professionals agree with my observation that the liver gets over-worked trying to sort, digest, and generally deal with an overload of un-needed, or un-absorbable supplements. (A congested liver will quickly affect all the other bodily functions.) In the beginning stages of illness we might feel a health improvement from the use of an arsenal of pills. But, since many of us are convinced that more is better, we keep on with a therapeutic dose of a supplement, instead of cutting back to a maintenance-level dosage, or eliminating certain supplements altogether.

There is no replacement for the intelligent use of foods for good health, as well as our best resource during times of illness. Two of the best books for well-documented information on the health giving properties of foods are: *Food Your Miracle Medicine* by Jean Carper and *Intuitive Eating* by Humbart "Smokey" Santillo, N.D. (see Recommended Bibliography). To sort through the labyrinth of supplements, from the traditional to the state-of-the-art, consult: *The New Nutrition: Medicine for the Millennium* by Dr. Michael Colgan (Ronkonkoma, NY: Advanced Research Press, 1994), and *Smart Drugs and Nutrients* and *Smart Drugs and Nutrients II*, both by Dr. Ward Dean, M.D. and John Morgenthaler (Menlo Park, CA: Health Freedom Publications, 1991).

FOOD COMBINING: THE BEST DIGESTIVE MIX

The degree to which we can properly digest and absorb our food (with their functional components) determines the value we get from those foods. Food combining can significantly help or hinder these processes. Poor combinations of foods within one meal can slow down or entirely disrupt proper digestion and absorption. On the other hand, the clever combining of foods within a meal can dramatically improve these processes.

For more comprehensive advice about food combining see *Intuitive Eating* by Humbart "Smokey" Santillo, N.D., (Prescott, AZ: Hohm Press, 1993), from which the following food combining chart (figure 1.2) was adapted, with permission. Don't get confused if, now and then, you read suggestions in *10 Essential Foods* which seem to conflict with this chart. This chart is meant as a very generalized beginning, and there are always healthy exceptions. Also, the foods mentioned in each category on the chart are examples of that category/type. Each category (for instance High Starch Foods And Vegetables) includes a huge variety of items. The examples are there just to get you started!

The basics of food combining within any given meal are:

1. Eat fruits only with other fruits. This means you may have an entire meal that is a cornucopia of fruits. For example: blend up pineapple juice and several different fresh fruits (like bananas, blueberries, peaches) with a few frozen strawberries for a wonderful breakfast or snack. For the best "digestive mix," avoid eating fruits along with milk products, proteins, vegetables, or any other foods. The eating of fruits (unless fruits are the meal) should be done at least 20 minutes before a non-fruit meal; or you should wait at least 45 minutes after a non-fruit meal before consuming your fruit.

2. When eating protein foods, whether animal- or plant-based, eat only one "type" at any given meal. For example, nuts and seeds (including Almonds), fish, dried beans, eggs—each of these would be a "type."

3. In combination with protein foods, eat a good quantity of fresh salad or other raw vegetables and/or cooked low starch vegetables such as dark-green leafy greens of all sorts, Broccoli (or any cruciferous vegetable) or Carrots.

4. Avoid protein foods combined in a meal with sugary foods or heavy starchy vegetables such as potatoes, pasta or winter squash. An exception to this (I know it is contrary to some health gurus) is that whole Brown Rice (*not* de-germed white rice) combines well with protein foods. Examples of this beneficial "mix" include: fish with Brown Rice; or Almonds (or other seeds such as sunflower or sesame) with Brown Rice.

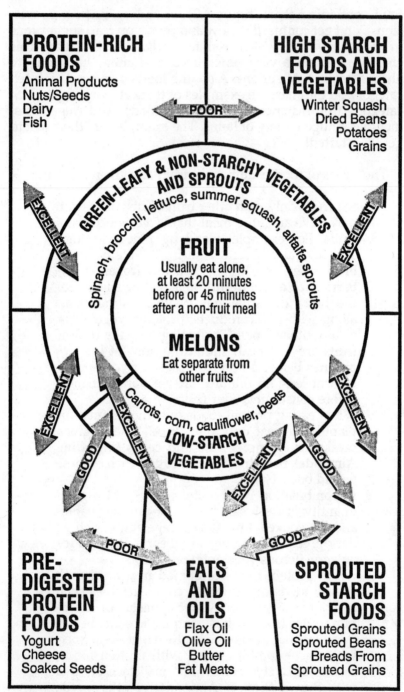

figure 1.2 Food Combining Guidelines

5. Most all vegetables combine well together, whether high or low starch, leafy-green or not, etc. I often make an entire meal out of a variety of vegetables. For example, one of my favorite meals is baked potatoes, along with a large colorful salad that includes Sprouts. On the food-combining chart (figure 1.2), this is partially indicated by having many types of vegetables listed around the entire inner circle of the chart. Variety is the key here.

THE CASE FOR ORGANIC FOOD

You may enter the Fresh Produce section of your local grocery store with the best of intentions, only to find your choices limited to unnaturally ripened, immature vegetables and fruits. Since these items have not been allowed to reach their full potential "on the vine," they did not get a chance to build the mature spectrum of functional components which you need for optimal nutrition. To add insult to injury, many fruits and veggies are "preserved" by a coating of wax or oil—substances which may be "OK'd" by the FDA, but which many food experts have determined are definitely toxic. (See: David Steinman and Samuel S. Epstein, M.D., *The Safe Shopper's Bible* New York, NY: Macmillan, 1995).

There are alternatives to such questionable produce, however. Fruits and vegetables which have been labeled "Certified Organic" are usually the most nutritious (even if they aren't as shiny). Produce from a neighborhood garden that you know is organic, yet is not officially certified, should never be overlooked. Indeed, you are fortunate if you have such a source at your disposal.

With organic produce you can be more certain that the foods you eat have been grown without the use of poisonous chemicals, such as herbicides and pesticides. These poisons can build up in the tissues of the body causing all sorts of health difficulties (and a health professional might not associate your symptoms with your regular ingestion of those chemicals, since fruits and vegetables supposedly contain minute or "safe" amounts). The public is often misinformed. Government agencies declare that certain agro-chemicals are only present at safe levels. Nonetheless, for years nutritional researchers have warned us that pesticide poisoning from eating contaminated foods leads to the breakdown of the immune system, and results in seemingly unrelated conditions such as weakened eyesight, skin eruptions, and more serious illnesses. I have seen a chronic skin rash, that nothing seemed to help, simply disappear when the person switched to organic foods, or eliminated a single contaminated food source, such as cherries from an orchard sprayed with pesticides. To my amazement, an unsprayed variety of the same food often agrees with the person perfectly.

In addition to being free of pesticides, herbicides and unbalanced fertilizers, my students agree that organic produce often has a better flavor and seems more satisfying to eat. For instance, many unofficial but persistent produce samplers, myself amongst them, find that it takes much less of an organic produce item to satisfy the palate than its agro-chemical-soaked counterpart.

Organic Foods (and the methods used to grow them) result in:
- *Continual replenishment* of the optimal nutritional content of our soils without the environmentally-destructive effects of poisonous farming methods. Mineral-rich food can only be grown on mineral-rich soils. (See more about the miraculously health-building nature of minerals in the Dulse Chapter.)
- *Measurably higher nutritional content* in our foods, including the entire spectrum of functional components. For example, at Rutgers University, organically grown food was found to be considerably richer in minerals, particularly trace minerals. Organic tomatoes had five times more calcium, twelve times more magnesium, three times more potassium and sixty times more manganese! Because of this higher nutritional content, a consumer often experiences a desire for less food.
- *Noticeably-enhanced flavors, textures and aromas* of foods.
- *No toxic, disease-producing and/or unbalanced substances,* such as pesticides, herbicides, fungicides, synthetic fertilizers and preservatives in our foods and soils which end up in our bodies as well.

A Detoxifying Solution

I don't know a single person who would rather be eating the impoverished foods offered in our produce markets instead of organic produce. However, for many consumers the availability and expense of organic foods is the prohibitive issue.

Fear not! I have found a solution that works for me, which I gladly pass along. I buy organic produce when the price is within my budget, and I grow my own food as much as I can. In addition to this, however, I do buy produce that is not organic. In either case, though, I soak produce for twenty minutes in what I call my "disinfecting detox-soak solution," which is a way of lessening the amounts of pathogens on those foods. Additionally, for non-organic produce, I employ a "detox-wash" for lessening pesticide and preservative residues. Refer to Chapter 2 where my "detox" processes are detailed step by step.

*** *** ***

With these simple nutritional basics in mind, the rest of the 10 Essential Foods system will be easier to understand and more enjoyable for you to investigate. In Chapter 2, I try to set the context for an entire relationship to food, food preparation, and eating. Have fun!

2

10 ESSENTIAL GUIDELINES
FOR FOOD SELECTION, PREPARATION AND CONSUMPTION

This chapter consists of lessons in lifestyle enhancement. With these guidelines you can confidently turn yourself into a hawk-eyed, sharp-minded, lightening-reflexed *food ninja, apprentice.* Your reward for such training will be improved health overflowing within you.

GUIDELINE 1: Relax! Eat All You Want! It's Guilt Free!

With the *10 Essential Foods* system and the principles it embodies, it becomes easy to relax and enjoy the entire "food arena" of life. With this system it is almost impossible to make a bad decision when faced with the often anxiety-producing food questions such as—what to eat, when to eat, how much to eat, and whether to eat anything at all! When your refrigerator and pantry are stocked with the huge variety encompassed within the *10 Essential Foods*, their Additions, Alternatives, and the 10 Essential Snacks (see Appendix C), you can confidently ask these "food questions" without a feeling of restraint and without thinking that you must surely lock the refrigerator for your own good! Especially if you are a person whose "food anxiety" sometimes revolves around "getting enough" you will be especially happy to learn more about what it can mean to "eat all you want" using these healthy foods.

"Simple is better," would be a good motto to apply to your general daily fare, but never let this approach stand in your way when proper feasting is in order! If I were invited to a *10 Essential Foods* feast for a special occasion, I might be disappointed if I were presented only with raw vegetable sticks, a pile of Sprouts, and steamed greens—even if I could eat all I wanted! I would certainly be looking forward to the magnificent and delectable display of incredible variety, from raw to cooked, sauced to marinated, simple to complex, of which *10 Essential Foods* is capable. For these occasions one would certainly go all out with a presentation that could include the *10 Essentials*, the Healthy Additions and the 10 Essential Snacks. And, for those rare and exceptional occasions we shouldn't hesitate to add a "heart's desire" selection from that secret list in our minds. The *10 Essential Foods* System is about saying "Yes!" to the huge variety of foods embodied in its basic principles and the magical and endless ways to present them. (See the Recommended Bibliography for Cookbook suggestions.)

A Word About Dieting

I am often asked if *10 Essential Foods* is a weight loss diet. The answer to this is "No, definitely not!" and "Yes, it certainly can be!" I prefer to think of it as a weight *balancing* way of relating to food. While it is entirely possible to lose or gain weight, depending upon your use of the *10 Essential Foods*, there is no deprivation in this system when choosing foods intelligently. For instance, most students tell me that they automatically lose weight by the simple act of replacing their habitual pre-packaged, processed, high fat and highly cooked foods with abundant quantities of the *10 Essential Foods*, (along with their Healthy Additions and the 10 Essential Snacks). Even if they are eating an ounce of healthy raw Sprouts or sunflower seeds every day, along with three or four tablespoons of Flax oil, both higher in calories than the other foods, the weight still drops off. I believe a person's weight-balancing metabolism can be repaired with these highly restorative foods. On the other hand, if you wanted to gain weight or get extra protein and calories for some reason, as a pregnant friend of mine recently did, it is not hard to do with the use of the tasty "seed balls" I describe in the KIDS LOVE THIS section of the Almonds chapter and/or by eating extra servings of the healthy oils I describe in the Flax Oil chapter. Animal foods will generally contribute to weight gain, so check out the healthy way to use them in chapter 13.

Eat All You Want . . . Within Reason!

Of course, this "eat all you want" philosophy, mentioned first in the Introduction, should be further elaborated as "eat-all-you-want-as-long-as-it-makes-you-feel-good." In other words, *some* common sense should apply.

TASOLE: Take the case of Tom. He fell in love with Flax Oil to the extent that he downed a half cup or more a day, on various foods, and then wondered why his bowel movements were a little oily, even though he felt great!

Lalitha says: I guess *you* can't digest that much oil Tom; but you're feeling great and that's a good sign. You may find that, over time, your desire for Flax oil may moderate as your need for its specific nutrients lessens. Also, look up Dr. Budwig's book on Flax oil in the Recommended Bibliography. Anyone who loves Flax oil like you do will be interested in what she has to say.

Take the case of Kathryn. She ate raw Almonds in amounts greater than she could properly digest (handfuls) and then called me with the worst intestinal gas experience of her life.

Lalitha says: Well Kathryn, what can I tell you? It will pass. Double-check that you were eating *raw* Almonds and not roasted or salted ones. In the future try eating just two or three Almonds at a time; and chew them very well. Wait awhile before you eat more and you will begin learning the best amount for yourself. Then, when you are doing the "eat all you want" plan, with your new education regarding amounts for yourself, you'll probably want less. Right? Eat all you want ... but want less. See how that works?

Here is the case of Anser who ate all he wanted of Carrots day in and day out—which turned out to be a pound of raw Carrots a day—and his skin became a pale orange color ... and then a *bright* orange color. He called me because he was having an unemployment problem.

Lalitha says: Look Anser. No wonder you are always unemployed! Do you think anyone in his right mind will hire an alien-appearing, orange-skinned computer nerd? Don't worry though, the orange color isn't permanent and doesn't indicate approaching death, or internal damage, although you might want to eat less Carrots and more of the other stuff recommended in this book. It's simply that your body is getting more than it thought possible of the orange phytochemicals (probably beta carotene) from raw Carrots. Yes, I know I say "eat all you want," but *Get a Life!* I mean it!

GUIDELINE 2: Cook Less For More Health

Without question, raw, properly harvested fruits and vegetables are the #1 powerhouses for health, especially if they are organic. Aim towards eating a minimum of 50% raw food every day. Since the majority of the American diet is built around cooked and processed foods, this goal of greatly increasing our raw/fresh food intake should be approached in the slow and steady fashion I describe in the Introduction. Many factors, such as body type and emotional disposition, the circumstances surrounding mealtime, the season of the year, the overall climate, etc., influence the incorporation of more raw foods into the diet.

Simply cooking your vegetables less, or eating a larger variety of whole foods in general, whether cooked or not, will notably increase your intake of lively functional components. While cooking does destroy functional components in fresh fruits and vegetables, a lot depends on the style and duration of the cooking method employed. Some foods *need to be cooked* for best digestive results. A few components seem to enhanced by *light cooking*, such as the wonderful beta-carotene. Whole grains and legumes of all sorts (i.e., dried beans, split peas, lentils) need to be well-cooked to get heightened nutrition and digestibility. Sea vegetable preparation depends on the type, but in general they can all be cooked without much loss of their fabulous mineral content.

In an article entitled "Beyond Vitamins" (*Newsweek*, April 25, 1994), author Sharon Begley interviewed many nutrition experts and reported on the stability of nutrients and phytochemicals under cooked and uncooked conditions. She learned that P-coumaric acid and chlorogenic acid, two phytochemicals that can stop the formation of cancer-causing substances and which are found in many fruits and vegetables (including Carrots), are not damaged by cooking. Begley further mentioned that sulforaphane, a cancer-preventing phytochemical found in Broccoli, does not seem to be destroyed with cooking.

Despite these reports, however, the majority of other bio-active functional components in the *10 Essential Foods*, such as vitamin C, delicate enzymes, or the important indoles in Broccoli can be lessened or, depending on the style and dura-tion of the cooking method, totally destroyed by heat.

Keep in mind that other factors can destroy the optimal nutrition in fresh foods even more than cooking does. Harvesting methods which favor unripe foods, growing in nutrient-depleted soil, heavy use of chemicals and fertilizers, improper handling or storing of produce—these factors also play an important role when determining the nutritional value of fresh foods.

Water Sauté Is In! Fried Foods Are Out!

Everyone knows (don't they?) that eating fried foods on a regular basis is a nasty habit. Fried foods are full of rancid oils and trans-fatty acids, among other things, which can quickly ruin your health. This is why I say that frying pans are obsolete. My frying pans have all now become water/herb "steam-sauté" pans; and I add oil to my food *after* cooking it to get the rich flavor I like.

Some food enthusiasts insist that using olive oil for a minute or two of quick, low heat stir-fry is not health damaging, and I must admit I am on the fence about that question. Although I don't do it myself, I definitely agree that if one *must* fry, the quick stir-fry I just described is far better than the deep-fry done in one of those horrible oils commonly used in restau-rants, as well as in many household kitchens.

For your inspiration here is my approach.

Lalitha's Water-Herb Sauté Method

1. Chop desired vegetables and gently place in a non-aluminum water-sauté pan (this used to be your frying pan), or into a non-aluminum wok. See Choosing Utensils, below.
2. Add desired cooking herbs and a small amount of water—just enough water to have it quickly come to a boil, steam away as the vegetables cook, and be almost totally gone by the end of this process. (Until you develop a system for

your particular pan, start with perhaps 1/8 inch of water in the bottom of the pan. Remember that almost all types of vegetables will release some of their natural liquid as they are sautéing. Many cooks like to add an even smaller amount of water to start with, adding tiny amounts of water or liquid seasonings such as soy sauce during the process in order to not end up with extra liquid in the end. The aim is to have vegetables which are naturally moist and still a little crunchy.)

3. On medium-to-high heat, bring vegetables, herbs and water to a boil.

4. Alternate between covering the pan for a minute or two (to enhance the steam-sauté process), and uncovering and gently stirring for a couple of minutes, until the vegetables are seasoned. These alternating steps may be repeated once or twice. Finish off with a light tossing/stirring of the uncovered vegetables until any remaining water is totally steamed away. (The entire cooking process may take no more than 5-to-10 minutes. Thus you end up with vegetables that are perfectly tossed, seasoned, steam-sautéed, non-soggy, still lightly crunchy and full of nutritional value.)

5. If desired, healthy oils (like unrefined Flaxseed, olive, sesame, or sunflower; see the Healthy Additions information in the Flaxseed Oil chapter) are now added after this water-herb sauté process is complete. This way you get the health-positive effects of the proper oils your body needs, without the health-negative effects of having cooked them! While I love the rich flavor that the oils, with the proper herbs, give in the recipe, added oil is not essential for wonderful flavor.

Avoiding Extremes

I am far from advocating a fanatical "eat-all-your-food-raw" attitude. Especially for people with poor digestive power, or those "in transition" who much prefer cooked foods, the process of light steaming (so that veggies still have a gentle crunch), the quick sauté with mostly water and herbs (as described above), or baking/roasting of vegetables or some fruits, loosens and gently softens the tough vegetable fiber where many nutrients and phytochemicals are trapped and makes these components more available for digestion.

In addition, the pleasure of eating is a crucial factor. Maybe we simply adore roasted Carrots and abhor eating them raw.

Our reticence to eat primarily raw food may be because we have weak teeth, or no teeth—there are endless variables at play here. The pros and cons of whether to cook or not to cook continue on and on.

Here are my own "bottom lines" on the cooking question:

1. Start with the best quality food you can get and store it properly.
2. Develop the life-positive habit of eating raw fruits and vegetables as often as possible, starting with small amounts, and aiming for at least 50% raw food every day.
3. Invent dips and sauces to enhance the attractiveness of eating fresh, raw fruits and veggies, if you like.
4. Cook foods simply, trying to maintain optimal nutrition, yet keeping in mind what is pleasurable for you. The amount of cooking might be along the lines of: cucumbers, not at all; Carrots, raw or steamed; Rice and beans, well-cooked; potatoes, anywhere from raw to baked but never fried.

Are you getting the idea?

GUIDELINE 3: Support Sensory Appeal

Cephalic regulation is the name for an important process that goes on in our bodies/brains relating to the sensory appeal of food. Both science and our own personal experience attest that the sensory appeal of food makes a big difference in the digestion and therefore absorption of nutrients from that food.

Suppose we took several of the *10 Essential Foods* and presented them beautifully: imagine Fig slices sprinkled with fresh lemon juice and a bit of fresh mint; Dulse; Sprouts, marinated in a delightful garlic, mushroom and herb dressing, and perfectly seasoned Brown Rice pilaf with water chestnuts. Just looking at the plate our mouths are watering in anticipation. This food has high sensory appeal and our cephalic regulation is encouraging us to take it in, to absorb this nourishment. Now, to make an extreme and cartoonish example for illustrative purposes, imagine further that a well-meaning food maniac armed with a blender turns that gorgeous plate of food into a "health drink." While this presentation may have the identical nutritional content in a glass as it did when sitting upon a plate, it would certainly be extremely low on the sensory appeal scale. While we might force ourselves to drink this meal down, convincing ourselves of its superb nutritional balance, our cephalic regulation, as the monitor of sensory appeal, might be resisting its uptake, discouraging the absorption or digestion of the nutrients it contains, no matter how many functional components were available. Cephalic regulation, therefore, becomes important in our food choices and in the question of "to cook or not to cook."

On the other hand, I know that a majority of us often determine sensory appeal based upon unhealthy, even self-destructive, psychological habits, many of which have been ingrained in us since childhood and strongly reinforced through television advertising. Our cephalic regulation itself may be somewhat "broken"; our determination of sensory appeal, off balance. Therefore, while keeping in mind that cephalic regulation does play a role in getting optimal nutrition from the foods we eat, it should not be used as an excuse to continue in self-destructive dietary habits which ruin our health, leading to premature aging, ill health and untimely death. I have found that for many people, developing skill and diversity in using the *10 Essential Foods* leads automatically to a more balanced cephalic regulation and more life-positive habits in general.

Health-Positive Sensory Appeal Can Be Learned by Anyone . . . or Enhanced.

Anyone can redirect a passion for cooking into developing a passion for proper seasoning and simpler, less-cooking-time methods by using herbs for flavor and inspiration, and learning healthy substitutions for less-healthy favorite foods of the past.

Two "must have" companion books to *10 Essential Foods*, especially for those transitioning from a diet of highly processed or pre-packaged foods to the *10 Essential Foods* system, or for those needing new inspiration for extraordinary and life-enhancing recipes, are: *Junk Food to Real Food* by Carol Nostrand (New Caanan, CT: Keats Publishing, 1994) and

Intuitive Eating by Humbart "Smokey" Santillo, N.D. (Prescott, AZ: Hohm Press, 1993). In Carol's book you will find instruction on a wide variety of food-related subjects—from setting up a properly organized "eating healthy" kitchen and proper choosing and handling of foods, to identification of the wonderful yet unfamiliar foods which are sold at health food stores. To top it off, the book contains over 250 delicious recipes! It is easy to get away from "cooking food to death" when you have a resource like Carol's book.

Use Carol's book or other resources (see: Cookbooks, in the Recommended Bibliography) to learn about zesty sauces and dressings made from miso (a salty or sweet tasting soybean paste of several varieties), herbed vinegars, ground sesame seeds or Almonds, etc., which are added to foods after a simple and short cooking. Investigate condiments that you decide are in line with the *10 Essential Foods* principles, such as pickled vegetables, mustard, mayonnaise made from cold-pressed canola oil, salsa and many others (see Appendix B). Carol even includes complete instructions for growing your own Sprouts, which goes hand-in-hand with my chapter on Sprouts. Keeping these ideas in mind, almost anyone will gain increasing enthusiasm for all the ways to use and present the *10 Essential Foods* while lessening the cooking time and thereby preserving more of the optimal nutritional content.

Santillo's *Intuitive Eating* takes you step by step, stage by stage, from wherever you are starting from to a healthier diet, with thorough discussions of all the whys and wherefores along the way. Sample menus with recipes are included.

GUIDELINE 4: Disinfect and Detoxify Your Fresh Foods— Organic as Well as Non-Organic, Plant-Source as Well as Animal-Source

As I briefly mentioned at the end of Chapter 1, I use a detoxifying solution with my non-organic as well as organic fresh produce. (Of course, if you have grown your own produce, or meats, there is less need for this process.) Here's a story to introduce you to this priceless procedure for fruits and vegetables; and see Chapter 13, about Meat, Fish, Poultry and Dairy for more background about why to do this detoxifying and disinfecting process for flesh foods.

TASOLE:

"Lalitha, how do you afford to buy all this wonderful organic produce?" Rachel observed while eating a meal at my house. "Whenever I eat over here the produce tastes so much livelier and crisper. I have a stronger sense of satisfaction with less of it, even though our preparation methods are quite similar. Your food just seems more potent; I can't quite describe what it is exactly, but I guess it's because yours is organic."

"It's probably from her garden," put in Rachel's husband Dan. "Right, Lalitha?"

"Not a bit," I said. "In fact, I think tonight's food all came from the same commercial food store where Rachel and I usually shop. But [I smiled cleverly], there *is* one secret little process I always use. If you promise to try it out for yourself, I'll tell you the whole deal."

I can almost always start Dan on a long string of guessing if I mention I have a secret method of any sort, so he started right off with: "I bet you have an electric gadget that puts out a frequency to preserve fresh foods better; no, no, wait! I have it. You have an herbal concoction of some sort that you spray on it all." (I suspect this last idea came from the fact that I am an herbalist.)

"OK. Are you willing to agree to try the process or not?" I asked them with a big grin. I knew I *had* them.

"Absolutely," they both said. Then, of course, Dan added, "I mean absolutely unless the gadget is too expensive or something."

"Here is the secret," I continued, unperturbed. "Whatever produce I bring home, *whether it is organic or not,* gets soaked for about twenty minutes in an organic, non-toxic disinfecting solution that eliminates significant amounts of parasites, parasite eggs, and pathogens such as fungus, bacteria and viruses, at least from the surface of the foods. In addition to this, to complete the detoxifying process for *non-organic* foods, I often scrub them with a special non-toxic, biodegradable "soap" to help remove some of the pesticide and preservative residues."

"Pathogens? What pathogens? They're farming with viruses now?" asked Rachel with mock seriousness in her voice.

"It's not hard to figure out at least one source of pathogens," I responded. "I'm sure you have regularly seen people in grocery stores sneezing and wheezing on the fresh produce. [I tried to be tactful and not get too graphic here. I knew Dan had a queasy stomach.] That happens at any type of store. Pathogens and parasite contamination on foods are a "given" in dealing with fresh foods, and they are air-borne as well as being transferred through handling. Added to this, non-organic produce is frequently covered with wax, oil or other stuff sprayed on as a preservative after harvesting, to say nothing of the pesticides and synthetic fertilizers used in farming ... well you get the picture. Whether organic or not, the produce gets my disinfecting soak and the non-organic produce often gets the additional wash. What you are noticing about my vegetables is the result of this process."

"So, where's this solution?" Rachel asked as she looked around the kitchen. "Do you make it yourself?"

"It's in that little bottle on the counter," I explained, pointing. "The magic formula is a thick, clear liquid; an extract of Grapefruit seed and pulp. I get it from the health food store; the brand I use is NutriBiotic®. For the "detox" process I mix 10-20 drops (depending on how contaminated I guess the food may be) with each gallon of cold water in a plastic dish tub. I give the water a quick stir because the Grapefruit extract is sticky and sticks to the bottom of the tub. Then I put in the produce and let the whole thing "sit" for 20 minutes. After that I take the produce out and let it drip-dry on a clean dishcloth which I spread on my kitchen counter. Once it is relatively dry (thirty minutes will do it) I put the produce in the refrigerator. That's it! In some cases with non-organic produce, I use the additional wash I mentioned. Simple."

Rachel couldn't quite believe it. "So the only difference between the food we just ate here and the food I have at home from the same store is this "detox" process? You're sure this food is not from your garden, or the organic market?"

"I'm sure, and that's it!" I smiled. "I rarely tell anyone that I have done this to the produce, but you would be surprised how many people comment on the flavor, liveliness, and that intangible something about my food, whether it is organic to start with or not."

"Of course," I added, "I certainly *prefer* organic produce whenever I can get it. My "detox" process cannot cancel out any chemical residues stored inside the cells and fibers of the produce, nor does it restore the nutrition missing from foods grown in depleted soils. It's a great way to maximize your food power, though. Be sure to try it."

Disinfecting Detox-Soak for Fruits, Vegetables and Meats

Use for organic as well as non-organic produce and meats.

For Fruits and Vegetables:

Using liquid Grapefruit extract (I use Nutri-Biotic®, see Appendix B), mix 10-20 or more drops of the extract for each gallon of water. You can fill a large bowl, sink, or plastic washtub as desired. (I use a ten gallon tub and do four days' worth of produce at once.) Soak the produce for approximately 20 minutes, then set it out to drain on a clean cloth spread on your counter-top. Drain it long enough so that it remains only slightly damp and not wilted. Then package it for storage in your refrigerator.

Salad greens do best if spun in a salad spinner after this disinfecting soak and before storage; or if soaked and spun just before use. Remember that some fresh foods, such as yams or sweet potatoes, are treated with preservatives that can partially or totally come off in the soak water. This, along with the effects of the soaking itself, may leave the food vulnerable to quicker spoilage. If you notice quicker spoilage with a particular food after detoxing it, pay attention to only buy and detox the amount of produce which you will use within a few days.

For Meats:

Use the same process as outlined above except use 20-40 drops of the Grapefruit extract per gallon of soak water. Alternatively, you may find it convenient to use a spray, instead of a soak. Simply put this "meat-detox mixture" in a spray bottle and thoroughly spray fresh meats, letting them "sit" for 10-20 minutes before cooking. This spray mixture can be kept for at least a month at room temperature, ready for any disinfecting use, including spraying on countertops, cutting boards, or your own skin! See more information about why to disinfect meats in Chapter 13, Meat, Fish, Poultry and Dairy.

Along with the disinfecting detox-soak, I wash non-organic foods with non-toxic soap to lessen the amount of pesticides and preservative residues on the surface of foods. This detox-wash also comes in handy if you are in a hurry and can't take the time to do the entire detox-soak procedure described above; or perhaps you have such a small amount of food to "detox" that a detox-wash, instead of the soak, might be more convenient. Ask at your local health food store for a non-toxic soap, or try the "non-soap" liquid soap made by NutriBiotic®, which also contains their wonderful Grapefruit extract and which is perfect for the purpose.

GUIDELINE 5: Grow It or Buy It. Finding Fabulous Foods.

Imagine this: you come home from a day's work, pluck a few cherry tomatoes from the plant growing in a five-gallon tub in front of your window or under a fluorescent grow-light (these lights are available at most variety, home-supply, or garden stores), cruise by the basket of Sprouts growing on your kitchen counter, pull out a Carrot from a tub on the patio, and *voila!*—you have a fresh, vibrant and extravagant display of functional components ready to eat in your salad. Add a few other items from the *10 Essential Foods*, and you end up with a prize meal. With even the minimal space and quantity of production I just described, you can make a big difference in the quality of your diet. Grow some of your own food—even if this means a single jar or basket of Sprouts in your kitchen (see the Sprouts chapter), or a 12-inch strip of lettuce in your window box.

Even a small windowless room has possibilities for an indoor garden; all you need is a grow-light to bring fresh greens and some Sprouts to life. Come to think of it, I've grown Sprouts while camping in the wilderness, or on-the-road when traveling in a foreign country (see the Sprouts chapter for a story about this). From my vast experience I can testify that there are few valid excuses for not growing something!

With a minimum of "want-to," any food you grow yourself will have less contaminants and probably more functional components than double the amount of the same food bought in a store. Why? Because you can harvest and eat home-grown food immediately, and you have complete freedom to use organic methods as you wish.

For those fortunate enough to actually have a patio on which to place a few large buckets or containers, an outdoor garden, or a four foot by eight foot space anywhere in the sun, you are in the running for one of my newer "best finds." I am referring to year-round, outdoor gardening (under any weather conditions) with Solar Pods developed by Leandre and Gretchen Poisson, authors of *Solar Gardening* (White River Junction, VT: Chelsea Publishing Company, 1994). By building one or more of the 4 x 8 foot solar pods they describe, you can (as I do) grow vegetables of all sorts even when it is well below freezing; even with snow on the ground and cold winds blowing! Solar gardening is so enjoyable that, like me, most people just keep adding pods as space allows. (One friend of mine has a pod in a previously unproductive strip alongside her garage and a pod in her back yard as well.)

The book *Solar Gardening* includes precise instructions for building and operating these pods (it is really so simple I can hardly justify the word *operating*), plus instructions for growing a large variety of different vegetables within the pods, according to the season and the growing zone you live in. During my first pod-winter, I easily grew enough salad greens to give some away.

Shop With Your Eyes Open

In each chapter of *10 Essential Foods* I will tell you in simple terms how to recognize the most potent food for your food dollar, how to make the wisest compromise (which we often are faced with doing) given the choices at hand, and how to look for the danger signals while shopping that mean: "Don't even bother putting it in the bag."

First of all, get organic foods when you are able. However, whether produce is organic or not, don't buy wilted Broccoli—or anything else wilted or discolored for that matter. Organic produce that is old or partly spoiled is simply old, spoiled produce—nothing esoteric about it. If you get seriously interested in the optimal nutritional content of foods, you should definitely start asking questions about when a food was harvested and how long it's been stored, etc.

The word *fresh* when applied to produce is extremely deceptive, since it emphasizes only a part of the picture. Only when a plant is allowed to come to maturity will it develop its full and potent complement of phytochemicals, enzymes, vitamins, minerals, and other bio-active substances. With phytochemicals and their fabulous potential for health and healing, this is especially important. (One signal whereby a plant knows to start creating certain phytochemicals is the maturation of its seed; this is particularly true with fruits.) To describe this optimal nutritional potential, the concept of *plant ripened* must be added to the concept of *fresh* in our education about foods in general, and about the *10 Essential Foods* specifically. (Exceptions to this "fully mature" idea include Sprouts and young wheat grass, which both have exceptional phytochemicals present in their infancy stages.)

To restate this important point I will repeat that we want *fresh, plant-ripened, organic produce* whenever possible. We want fruits and vegetables with maximum health-power for humans to enjoy.

If these concepts are somewhat new to you, you may be wondering how to get started. After all, as a friend recently pointed out, "Listen, Lalitha, my next shopping trip is tomorrow!"

OK. Right. Here's where some simple and easy-to-learn skills come into play.

TASOLE: "The object of this 'shopping game,' " I said to Sue as she headed off to buy the day's produce for our Whole Foods Seminar, "is to get the best quality for the best price, given the choices available. Please pay attention to details. Carefully look through the stacks of produce and pick out the best specimens—unwilted, unbruised, uncoated with waxes or oils if possible, ripe. Look for in-season specials, and if there is organic produce that looks good for the price be sure to give that precedence over the regular stuff."

Since I do tend to be overly bossy about a few things, Sue became impatient near the end of my instructions and rushed out the door with a laugh, saying, "Right, right. I know what to look for."

When she returned, the class gathered for the pleasurable ritual of looking over each day's cornucopia with the shopper. We began to fill up the "detox tubs," into which we were placing all the fresh food.

"Give me the prepackaged produce—yes, that Broccoli and those Carrots—to open and check," I called out to a student. I began to open the Carrot package and undo the rubber band from the Broccoli stalks in order to check for "clinkers," as we called the produce that did not meet our specifications. Once unpackaged or unbanded, the wilt of the Carrots and Broccoli became obvious. When a student called out "Clinker" it was a sign to gather around for closer inspection. (We had a least one "Clinker" nearly every day in those seminars, as students learned the finer points of produce inspection.)

"Most of the fruits and vegetables look fantastic, Sue, but you've 'been had' here in the Carrot and Broccoli departments!" I chuckled. (No one ever took the "Clinkers" too personally. It was all a humorous part of our learning style.)

"Rats!" said Sue. (She didn't really say rats, but ... well, you know ... this is a family food book, that anyone might read and so ...) "I was sure they were good because the color seemed bright and they felt firm to me," Sue continued good-naturedly.

"It's the old 'tie-or-package-vegetables-together-and-they'll-brace-each-other-and-seem-crisper' story," I remarked, a bit sarcastically. "And look here, in the middle of the bunch of Broccoli—one clump is starting to spoil. In this case, we'll throw out the spoiled parts, detox the rest and eat them right away. No big deal."

Other "Clinkers" during that seminar were the apples that were kept shiny and crisp-seeming on the outside with wax, only to be mealy on the inside. There were the ultra-orange oranges (sprayed with coloring), which turned out to be dry on the inside, as compared to the greenish-tinged, uncolored oranges that were the juiciest we had tasted in a long time. (I was told by a produce manager that Florida oranges have a naturally greenish tinge when ripe, so they are sometimes sprayed with coloring to be uniformly orange with the California ones which don't naturally have the greenish tinge when ripe.) Yet another example were the green and sparky-looking alfalfa Sprouts (on top) which turned out to be spoiling terribly (on the bottom).

"How can we possibly know what all to check for?" Sue asked, with a bit of discouragement. "How do we know how long an apple has been waxed; when it was harvested; or what's in the middle of prepackaged produce?" She summed up her mood by saying, "Maybe we are just being too picky."

Upon hearing this last phrase, Gladys, the oldest person in the class (at sixty-eight years), took things firmly in hand. "No! Never too picky! It just takes continued experience, Sue, and then your eye and your touch just knows!" Gladys went on to explain, "I learned so much from the produce manager at my store on how to choose the best foods. Some produce managers really know what's what. Of course, I don't think they are going to come up to a customer and say, 'You know, those apples are from last season and won't be that tasty on the inside.' But, let me tell you, these managers usually love to talk about any details having to do with their produce. If you come right out and ask about the apples, for instance, they'll most likely tell you. When I ask Ron, he's my produce man, 'When were these apples harvested?' or 'How do I pick out the best cantaloupe?' or 'Were these tomatoes picked green and ripened with gas?' or 'How can I best ripen this fruit at home?' he knows it all. In fact, it was Ron who told me, 'Sniff the end of a cantaloupe to tell its quality and ripeness instead of squeezing it ... Move the produce around within a loosely prepackaged bag, like with carrots, citrus, apples, and potatoes, to make sure they aren't wilted, or soft, or spoiling in the middle ... Put unripe produce in a brown paper bag with some green bananas. The gas given off by the ripening green banana will ripen the other produce.' It sure was an eye-opener when I began asking him when certain things were harvested, what they were coated with, or whether they were colored, etc."

We always enjoyed it when Gladys told us things she had learned over the years. She ended up her small food lecture by saying again, "Never too picky! Don't even think it! We want lively, uncontaminated food and great health. Find a good produce manager, you'll see!"

I couldn't have agreed with her more.

GUIDELINE 6: Choose Utensils That Honor Your Food

There are many wonderful utensils, machines or gadgets which are hard to ignore and highly useful in food preparation, yet I can't say they are truly needed. Some good ideas along these lines can be found in Carol Nostrand's *Junk Food To Real Food*, as well as in some of the cookbooks listed in the Recommended Bibliography.

In choosing kitchen implements my basic rules for myself are that they must be highly practical, cost effective, and still allow for plenty of hands-on work with the food.

Nothing that comes into contact with any part of the food during preparation should be made of aluminum (that includes aluminum cookware and aluminum foils), or any of the other toxic materials I am about to write about. Aluminum is neurotoxic and can get into your food, especially with the heat of cooking. Toxic levels of aluminum in body tissues are increasingly being linked as a contributing factor in Alzheimer's disease as well as other illnesses. For more specifics on aluminum toxicity, consult the *The Safe Shopper's Bible* by David Steinman and Samuel Epstein, M.D., *The New Nutrition: Medicine for the Millennium* by Dr. Michael Colgan, and *Smart Drugs and Nutrients* by Ward Dean, M.D. and John Morgenthaler (see Recommend Bibliography).

Copper cookware can contribute toxic levels of copper to our bodies. Use copper cookware only if it is lined with stainless steel, and replace that lining when it wears thin.

Ceramics can contribute toxic levels of lead to food. Many sources, including the *The Safe Shopper's Bible* point out that this is especially true if the ceramic cookware comes from Italy, India, China, Mexico or Hong Kong. My educated guess is that ceramics in and of themselves are not the problem, but that the problem lies in lead-contaminated glazing compounds.

Use *The Safe Shopper's Bible* to identify sources of toxic metals and to help avoid these, and for specific information on alternatives to these and other health damaging substances commonly found in our households.

Gadgets and Machines for a Healthy Kitchen

The following list represents what I consider the basics for a healthy kitchen. I list specific manufacturers where necessary, especially in cases where I have wasted money on others until

I found "the one." If no specific source is listed, assume that many good ones are available and have fun shopping around.

- Wooden or stainless steel spoons and stirring "sticks."
- Stainless steel vegetable steamer.
- Stainless steel, glass, or black cast-iron pots and pans.
- Blender.
- Vegetable juicing machine. See Appliances in Supplies Appendix B.
- Well-stocked rack of cooking herbs.
- Non-aluminum dishes and eating utensils.
- Lettuce/leafy greens spinner (most indispensable of all for salad lovers, or "wanna-be" salad lovers!).

In addition to this short list, two good mail-order resources for health-positive small kitchen equipment and utensils of all sorts are:

1. Gold Mine Natural Food Company. 3914 Hancock Street, San Diego, CA. 92110-4307. Telephone 1-800-475-3663.
2. Kushi Institute. P.O. Box 7, Becket MA., 01223-0007. Telephone (413) 623-5741, extension 104.

GUIDELINE 7: Chew! It is Easy, Inexpensive, and Highly Profitable!

Chew your food excruciatingly well. Don't be like the adults who my healing class for kids observed. We found that most adults, almost 100% of the time, ate their foods somewhat hunched over their plates. They would give little more than a cursory chew to each quickly shoveled bite before they swallowed a huge mouthful at one time. These people weren't involved in a cross country race or anything, but your common, ordinary, harried and unconscious adult! Where did they all learn such health-denying habits? The children certainly learned a lot of what *not* to copy from these observations.

Chewing begins the major digestive action as foods are ground and mixed together with enzymes contained in saliva. In fact, the bioavailablity of several necessary components, such as sugars and starches, is severely limited if the chewing process is largely ignored. In addition, chewing is the primary activity for releasing some nutritional components, including phytochemicals, from the fibers of fruits and vegetables. Since the *10 Essential Foods* system emphasizes the use of raw or lightly-cooked vegetables and fruits (whose fibers need to be broken down), chewing becomes all the more significant.

Often, when I am asked for advice in improving digestion, I will simply suggest chewing food in smaller amounts and more thoroughly—a pertinent, highly effective, easily applied and inexpensive "therapy" for poor digestion. I am often disappointed, however, to find that most people, even to preserve their own health, resist chewing their food as stubbornly as if I were asking them to eat raw snake innards from a recent road kill!

On the other hand, I remember one particular student who, upon hearing me stress the attributes of chewing, set up a rule for herself of chewing each bite of food at least fifty times. Her commitment caused much comment and hampered her social style as she energetically chewed away, looking quite like a charming squirrel. Often she left the table long after everyone else had departed. Despite it all, she improved her previously poor digestion and became one of the most efficient "digesters" I've ever known. This upscale in digestive capacity led to greater absorption of nutritional components, which in turn led to wonderfully enhanced health, vitality and stamina. While I'm not suggesting that you make a "chew 50 for 1" rule for yourself (after all, how long does it take to chew applesauce, for instance), I can't state strongly enough the importance of chewing food thoroughly.

A teacher of mine once asked her students to chew a mouthful of bread until there was literally nothing left of it, to illustrate how completely certain foods can be digested solely in the mouth. In determining how much chewing is enough, I suggest that you chew until there are no dominant lumps in any particular mouthful, i.e., the smoother the consistency the better. Certainly, such chewing does take more time than most of us are used to; but, what the heck ... just eat less and chew more.

Remember the folk saying: "There are no teeth in your stomach!"

GUIDELINE 8: Educate Your Loved Ones Through Culinary Creativity and Enlightened Encouragement

You may like these *10 Essential Foods* ideas, but what about the rest of your family, or business-meal companions, or partner on a date? All these relationships call for a careful, non-pushy approach, unlike that of one new student who righteously reported: "I just announced to my family that I was only going to cook meat once a week from then on, and that I wasn't buying any more junk foods. They'll get used to it!"

I advocate a more creative and gentle approach, like the student who said: "My family agreed to participate in food investigations with me. We made it a game and each day or so I introduced a new food, or a new way of preparing an 'old' one. Then we would talk about whether we liked the food, or how to improve it. During these 'experiments,' I was always careful to also provide foods my family was used to, so that no one ever felt pressured."

In reading *10 Essential Foods* you will be learning many new health-enforcing concepts. If another member of your family, a friend, or someone you meet is interested in hearing what you are discovering, go ahead and share, with enthusiasm. But, if no one in your vicinity is intrigued by the topic of phytochemicals, antioxidants, or a major dietary upscale don't be discouraged; and don't wait to get started on your own food improvements.

For your own education, as well as that of your children, begin to develop a habit of only buying foods that contribute to good health. When you spend your food dollar on healthy foods, filling your refrigerator or food pantry with them, you don't have to put certain foods off-limits, but can confidently invite your family to "look around and see whatever you feel like eating today." This is a wonderfully easeful way to educate yourself and your children, and to train yourselves in choosing what your body needs for balance and satisfaction.

Because food tastes differ, refrain from making prejudgements on another's behalf about his or her potential preferences. When faced with an unfamiliar food or preparation technique, meet the challenge without sour facial expressions, or doubtful remarks such as, "You (I) probably won't like this, but you (I) should try it anyway." In the Dulse chapter, I tell a story of a child who was fascinated in seeing me eat Dulse, and so wanted to try some. The child's mother had grave doubts about it, and said so in front of the child. These unconscious remarks could have discouraged the child from ever trying Dulse, but happily in this situation the child went right ahead and ate it. Much to the mother's surprise, Dulse slowly became a desired household food.

Children should never be forced to eat foods they don't want to eat. Yet, at the same time, they can be invited (and enticed) into trying new foods when these items are presented properly. At the end of each chapter I include a section labeled KIDS

LOVE THIS. There I suggest food presentations that have usually been well-received by children (and adults) I have known. Start with these simple suggestions while you are developing your own ideas about how to encourage your children in healthier eating.

I look forward to mealtimes; and you should too. I never force myself to "tough-it-out" in eating particular foods solely because I learned that something was supposed to be "good for me." Food education is an education about life—and how to sustain it vibrantly, fully and with great enjoyment, for longevity. At the same time, this education is a process which requires at least a bit of retraining for many of us. It takes time to re-orient and re-educate our thinking and our habits. While initiating changes both for ourselves and other members of our family we should allow for plenty of transition time, reasonable compromises, and lots of creative alternatives as the process moves ahead. Avoid food arguments; encourage food adventures.

GUIDELINE 9: Make Food Your Best Health Support

I. The All-Vegetable Miracle Treatment

Whenever I feel the slightest twinge of an illness trying to settle in, I will often change to a diet of only vegetables (raw or lightly steamed), for a couple of days. This diet may or may not include fresh vegetable juices, miso broth and some sea vegetables (see MISO in Appendix B). Additionally, I often add an herbal antibiotic formula (such as those containing echinachea and goldenseal, or the Nutribiotic® mentioned in the Grapefruit chapter, or the Enhanced Garlic Formula described in my book, *Ten Essential Herbs*) when needed.

This vegetable-diet strategy temporarily takes the pressure off of my digestive system, allowing the body to fully attend to detoxifying itself, rebalancing, and strengthening the immune system. The concentrated but easy-to-digest functional components in the vegetables help the body fight off illness, usually within record-breaking time. Additionally, this diet brings a focused sense of well-being back into my body. I always find it far more potent to get this healing assistance from freshly prepared vegetables than from a pile of separate supplements of individual nutrients and phytochemicals. The vegetables themselves contain a great variety of synergistic components that you simply don't get in a supplement.

While I always advise the vegetables-only diet as the first choice for speeding recovery from common illness, or stress-induced physical symptoms, some people may want to take additional nutrients such as vitamin C tablets, or a trace mineral supplement. However, only add extra supplement tablets if you really experience that they help in your own case. While it is true that the right supplement (in the right amount, at the right time) can greatly enhance recovery from illness or stress, also remember that, especially when someone is ill, the liver (and therefore immune activities) gets easily overwhelmed with having to process too many supplements. When this happens, you may experience nausea or headache from the supplement overload; and you may be slowing down the recovery process rather than enhancing it. (You don't necessarily need professional help to figure this out, either. Often it is obvious when supplements are not agreeing with you.) Feel free to experiment with taking less supplements, or eliminating certain ones, during illness.

Remember, the vegetables-only diet has worked miracles for me, and for my friends! No reason that it can't do the same thing for you too.

II. The Unbeatable Lemon Body-Tonic

Fresh lemon is one of the Healthy Additions to Grapefruit in the *10 Essential Foods* system. And, a lemon-tonic can provide extraordinary help in general health maintenance, especially for those who have suffered from "foods abuse" in the past, those who travel, or people who work in "food-challenged" circumstances. A lemon tonic consists simply of the fresh-squeezed juice from one-half lemon, perhaps mixed with water.

For general tuning-up of your system, pick one day a week as your "lemon-tonic day," preferably the same day each week. Drink the tonic once or twice during that day. Also, on this day, eat only vegetables and drink at least two quarts of pure water (an ordinary daily minimum for good health) or herbal tea. (Fresh vegetable juices are wonderful additions on this day, but keep in mind that they count for food intake, not water or tea intake.)

Fresh lemon juice is famous for its ability to stimulate a congested liver and thereby stimulate the decongestion of other body functions. Many of my friends use this lemon-tonic process regularly, whether one day a week or once a month, with a noticeable improvement in vitality and strength. I highly recommend this procedure since it involves nothing extreme. Just a simple and effective tonic.

III. The Magnificent Mono-Diet (and Outright Fasting)

A mono-diet consists of eating just one special food, all day long, for one or more days, with the intention of giving the body an intensive rest and a further encouragement to cleanse itself. Foods often used for a mono-diet include watermelon, apples, plain Brown Rice, or one particular vegetable such as Carrots in whole and juice form. Mono-diets work quite well for many people, and are used in a similar way and for similar reasons as the vegetable-only diet.

Pick a fruit or vegetable that agrees with you especially well, and one that you can safely eat alone for one to five days. Many friends have done this for a few days every three months or so, as general health maintenance.

A mono-diet can be pursued for longer periods of time, in which case professional supervision is recommended.

True "fasting" is when you eat no food at all, while at the same time drinking plenty of pure water, usually at least three quarts a day. One quart of this water could be made into an herbal tea (try yarrow, or alfalfa with spearmint). Fasting is advocated by many health professionals for specific cleansing and healing purposes and is best undertaken with the supervision of a health professional.

Some people loosely use the word *fasting* when they really mean using a mono-diet, or drinking only fresh juices, or just eating simply. While each of these approaches has its own benefits, they are technically not true fasts. Some might even consider my vegetable-only diet in the category of fasting—which definition would be way off the mark! My own experience with fasting, coupled with my observation of others, has convinced me that fasting can be a powerful and sometimes dramatic tool for healing and rejuvenation.

IV. More Step-By-Step Healing Programs Using Whole Foods

Many good books will supply you with exact instruction on additional cleansing diets, use of fresh juices for health and fasting, or diets for special health conditions. See the Recommended Bibliography, and especially note *Intuitive Eating* and *Junk Food To Real Food*.

For medical supervision using whole foods for healing during serious illness, see the list of professional Clinics in Appendix A.

GUIDELINE 10: Practice Concious Undereating

Conscious undereating is a habit of never eating any meal to the point of feeling totally full; you simply stop eating well before you would feel "stuffed." I consider this such an important practice that if you only have patience or inspiration to try one Guideline this year, or ever, I would definitely recommend conscious undereating for its overall benefit to your health.

By conscious undereating I *do not* mean starving yourself! In fact, for some people, like those who need to gain weight, it may mean eating more, or at least more often. According to the guidelines of this art form, as well as the *10 Essential Foods* system in general, I still eat three meals a day (or more or less if I want to), even though I am a small person. The point is that I am conscious about what I eat and how much I eat at each meal. Conscious undereating allows *all* of your mealtimes (and snack times as well) to be deeply satisfying, highly enjoyable, and even quite "robust" occasions!

Conscious undereating is a rocketship ride to transformational changes in body, psyche and soul. In a positive way, this particular bit of fine-tuning shoots well past common sense and good health. (I know this is a big claim I am making, but I'm convinced of it.) Conscious undereating is partly a philosophy and partly an activity. As you discover and explore its many-faceted aspects in eating for health, longevity and profound rejuvenation, you literally start to practice a new, and high art form.

When eating a meal, many of us know when we have reached the point of *just beginning* to feel satisfied. If we pay attention, we can detect both a definite bodily sensation and a signal from the brain. Usually, however, most of us continue eating beyond this signal, to the point of feeling quite full, or even further to the point of being absolutely stuffed. Then, a few minutes later, the meal seems to have expanded in our stomachs and we feel fuller still!

If we *have* overeaten, that "few-minutes-later" phenomena can be a real killer—often with symptoms such as heartburn, nausea, gas, bloatedness, headache, dulled mental acuity, depression and lethargy ... to name a few. But, how can we (Americans especially) expect anything different from ourselves? To begin to discern the "minutes-before-comfortable-fullness" (let's call it the MBCF), and then to stop eating at that point (conscious undereating), goes completely against the eating habits we have practiced for a lifetime, and these habits have deep roots that extend into our emotional and psychological structure. *We want it all and we want it now!* (Remember, healthy foods can also be overeaten, as far as sheer amount is concerned. Your body may be all excited at the plethora of incoming functional components, only to go into shock when the true scope of the intake becomes apparent.)

Breaking these habits will provide a significant challenge to us as prospective *food ninjas*. But the efforts will be well-rewarded.

The art of conscious undereating can be broken down into three basic steps:

Step One, simply begin to recognize the MBCF, without feeling obligated to *do anything* about it at all. However long this discovery takes (whether minutes or months), training your attention to recognize this signal is the all-important place to start.

Step Two is to *occasionally* stop eating the instant you recognize the MBCF, even if you still have food on your plate ... even if you paid for a larger meal ... even if your Auntie hovers over you (perhaps in your imagination) saying, "Clean your plate," or "You need to eat more; eat, eat!" (Obviously it is easier to begin practicing Step Two at ordinary mealtimes, rather than on special holidays, family feasts or during times of high peer pressure.) Eventually, stopping at the MBCF becomes a more frequent occurrence. Finally, it becomes your spontaneous, constant, life-positive response at *all* meals.

Step Three, pause for a moment before putting any food into your mouth and simply ask yourself this question: "Will the eating of this food truly add to a condition of strength, health and well-being for me?" Then, listen for your answer, and act accordingly if you can (or at least be aware, without guilt, when you are not acting accordingly).

That's all there is to the basic *outward* practice of conscious under-eating (more about the *inward* activity coming). Admittedly, what I am suggesting is radical for most people to consider, perhaps even extreme, unthought of, shocking ... yet intriguing at the same time. If it sounds fairly simple in the way I am describing it, just try sustaining the practice of conscious undereating for any length of time and you'll see how deeply unsettling, yet transformative, the practice is. Remember, conscious undereating is a way of fine-tuning your intake of foods and nutrients on every level: physical, psychological and spiritual. This art form is for those who are committed to healthier life; those who support the basic ideas behind the 10 *Essential Foods* approach. Nonetheless, I caution you to begin as slowly as you need to. Think of conscious undereating as you would any art form, and don't expect to perform like Van Gogh, or Maria Callas or William Faulkner tomorrow.

Inwardly, conscious undereating invites you to develop skills of sensitivity, perception and attentiveness to both physical and other more subtle signals, along with the ability to act on them. Furthermore, the degree to which your physical system is efficiently handling the uptake and utilization of the functional components in foods will correspond in many ways with your increasing ability to efficiently handle subtle nutrients, such as affection, understanding and creative energy. For instance, to give one over-simplified example, when your liver is not continually overworked due to your overeating, or because it must sort out the poisons generated by contaminated foods, it has time and energy to produce miraculous "chemistries" (that's the best way I can describe this) which have to do with feelings of pleasure, mood stability, balanced temperament and clear, creative thinking. (There is actually a physical chemistry that corresponds to the ability to like yourself more. It's true!)

When both your inner and outer digestive systems are accustomed to the art of conscious under-eating, not dampened or benumbed by taking in more "food" than you can handle, you actually start accumulating a type of "digestive power," on every level. Then, when daily occasions arise where your fullest human potential is called for, you are more than ready; you are *spectacular*!

Without describing more of the transformational possibilities that await you (perhaps a subject for my next book), I will encourage you once again to pursue this fine art and discover for yourself what magic it can do. As you realize the startling differences this practice can make towards vitality, stamina and longevity in your "emotional," "intellectual," "psychological," and "spiritual" bodies, besides its effects on your physical body, you will be hooked on this fine art forever.

In my own case, I have pursued the art of conscious undereating for many years of my adult life and am still uncovering new and more subtle advantages of this multi-faceted approach to health and healing.

Conscious Undereating Has Immediate, Practical Benefits!

Whether or not you ever accept conscious undereating as an art form or spiritual practice, there are still great benefits to be had. Here are a few glimpses into the more immediate and practical benefits to be gained.

When MBCF (minutes-before-comfortable-fullness, remember?) are recognized and acted upon through the immediate cessation of eating, digestive functions are left in peak operational mode, perhaps better than you ever knew they could be, and feelings of strength, energy and well-being continue to *increase* after the meal is over. (Not decrease, as many of us have experienced under ordinary, less conscious eating conditions.)

Furthermore, since your body is not overwhelmed by the sheer magnitude of the digestive job which most of your meals require, it will be able to take the incoming functional components from the food and use them to move right ahead into rebuilding damaged tissues, repairing weak digestive functions, healing itself of long and short-term illness, and feeding crucial chemical processes such as energy, hormone, and enzyme production, to name just a few.

Conscious undereating is also practical good news for travelers, people who eat out a lot, those who don't eat as optimally as they prefer, and for the rest of us during holiday feasts of all types. If MBCF are acted upon, increased digestive "power" can become available even when eating foods that are "less than healthy." (Believe me, I have used this "power" to enjoy and easily assimilate all kinds of food under numerous compromising circumstances!)

Conscious Undereating: The Advanced Perspective

The best teacher of the healing arts I ever had emphasized the heightened potential for healing and for the body's production of "transformative chemistry" through the simple habit of eating absolutely nothing after about 5:30 P.M. each evening, except for water or a little fresh juice. She taught us that the body would then be signaled for the heightened production of endocrine "substances" and hormones, resulting in increased stamina, rejuvenation, healing and creativity.

Following my teacher's instruction I would eat a regular breakfast, then lunch, then perhaps an early, lighter meal for dinner as I trained myself to not eat past 5:30 P.M. Later, this process evolved into eating a nutritious and hearty brunch about 10 A.M. and then another substantial meal about 4 P.M., with perhaps a snack at 1 P.M. and/or some juice about 7 P.M. This two-main-meals-a-day-plus-a-snack plan became my preference, and formed the foundation for the larger process I began to call conscious under-eating.

Over the years I have learned about other healers, mystics, yogis and scientists who have studied this under-eating phenomena, or explored the benefits of eating nothing past late afternoon or early evening. In the November 25, 1996 issue of *Time* magazine, author Jeffrey Kluger, in his article "Can We Stay Young?" reported up-to-the-minute findings of scientific research from around the world on the subjects of longevity and aging. Many exciting breakthroughs were discussed, not the least of which being that eating less has been shown to increase the lifespan of rats by one-third, and for humans that would mean another thirty years! Molecular biologist George Roth of the National Institute on Aging in Bethesda, Maryland was one of the scientists involved in this particular longevity research. Roth is enthusiastic about these findings even though he points out that most Americans don't seem willing to eat less, even if it would gain them thirty years of life! Apparently, Roth is now conducting further experiments on the life-extending effectiveness of caloric restriction in primates and is quoted in the article as saying: "I think caloric restriction could take us beyond a life-span of 80, maybe even 120."

Roth is talking about eating approximately one-third less food than you presently do (these "guesstimates" refer to the average American's diet). For anyone seriously working with the *10 Essential Foods* system, you are *already* on the right track! The high-level art-form of conscious under-eating is much more far-reaching than simple caloric restriction. ("Caloric restriction" sounds more like the language of a usual "special diet," doesn't it?). Nevertheless, the possible addition of thirty (or more) years of vibrant health is a lovely side effect worth considering; one that should perk us up to pay serious attention to the principles involved in conscious undereating.

An interesting addendum to the subject: an Austrian friend recently wrote to me about the work of Dr. Johannes Huber of Vienna. Huber is both a theologian (former assistant to Cardinal Dr. König), and a gynecologist/hormone specialist.

Dr. Huber has done much research about melatonin, a hormone which is getting copious international publicity lately for its role in the sleep cycle, for help with jet lag, as a catalytic substance for enhanced functioning of the immune system, as well as for its anti-aging effects.

Since I often get clues to or confirmations about my own investigations through synchronistic communications from friends, I found her letter intriguing. She wrote:

> Dr. Huber is a great physician who does not prescribe drugs or do surgery unnecessarily and obviously leads a spiritual life. [*He says that*] there is no need to take melatonin pills, because there is a way to produce melatonin in a natural way; i.e., if you don't have dinner your life will be prolonged, because not eating in the evening produces additional melatonin. Drink only juices or herb teas in the evening. Otherwise have a regular breakfast and a regular lunch [*perhaps a late lunch as I described above*], and "leave the dinner to your enemies." [*Huber's words.*]
>
> Melatonin increases your well-being and it strengthens the immune system. Unfortunately not eating in the evening is asocial, because in the evening people get together to eat dinner! I keep this on my mind and whenever there is an opportunity to skip a dinner (or just eat an apple) I do it gladly. Even before melatonin became in vogue, it was well known that undereating in the evening makes you feel much better, but now that we know about melatonin, there is even more reason to do so.

* * *

The context for the rest of this book has now been set. These introductory chapters are your training manual. Refer back to them as often as you wish. With both nutritional data and these valuable Guidelines available, you are now ready to proceed on a ten-stop journey of enjoyment, interest and high adventure, as we travel to each of the remarkable planets in the *10 Essentials Foods* system.

ALMOND TORTE : Flour Free
(makes two 9" layers)

6 eggs, separated
1/2 cup honey
2 tsp. vanilla extract
1/4 tsp. almond extract
2 1/2 Tbs. lemon juice <u>and</u>
1 1/2 Tbs. lemon peel (1 lemon)
1/4 cup cooked baking potato (about 3 oz. potato, skinned, diced, simmered and cooled in cold water to room temperature)
2 cups ground unblanched almonds (1 1/2 cups unground. Grind 1/3 cup at a time.)

Preheat oven to 350°

Prepare two 9" cake pans: Butter the bottoms but not the sides of the pans. Line the bottoms with brown paper or parchment paper, cut to fit. Don't butter the paper.

In a large bowl, beat the egg yolks with an electric mixer until they are thick and lemon colored (about 6 minutes). Add the honey, a small amount at a time, beating another 15 minutes. Add the lemon peel, juice, and extracts; then add the 1/4 cup potato, and mix again.

Add the ground almonds, a small amount at a time, mixing them in very well.

In a separate large bowl, beat the egg whites with an electric mixer until the whites form soft peaks, but are not dry. Gently fold the whites into the batter.

Bake 40 to 50 minutes at 350°. Let the cake cool in the pan on a wire rack before removing. (It will fall slightly.) Then, carefully loosen the torte from the sides with a knife, and remove. Let cool before serving or adding icing.

Serve as is, or add icing.

Recipe from: Nostrand, Carol. *Junk Food to Real Food* (New Caanan, CT: Keats Publishing, 1994, p. 260.) Used with permission.
For another great almond treat see the Almond Seed Ball recipe at the end of this chapter.

FUNCTIONAL COMPONENTS
In 100 Grams of Almonds, Raw, Shelled, Unblanched (light brown inner skin still in place):

Serving Size: 1 oz. (28.4 grams, or approximately 15-20 almonds), unroasted, unsalted, unanythinged! These almonds are the type commonly found in bags or bins at stores and sold as "raw."

Calories	589.0
Protein	19.95 g
Fat	52.21 g
Carbohydrates	20.4 g
Fiber	2.71 g
Cholesterol	0
Calcium	226.0 mg
Phosphorus	520.0 mg
Magnesium	296.0 mg
Potassium	732.0 mg
Sodium	11.0 mg
Iron	3.66 mg
Copper	0.942 mg
Manganese	2.273 mg
Zinc	3.0 mg
Selenium	2.8 mcg
Chromium	yes
Boron	2.2 mg
Vitamin A	0
Vitamin C	.6 mg
Vitamin B1 (Thiamin)	.211 mg
Vitamin B2 (Riboflavin)	.779 mg
Vitamin B3 (Niacin)	3.361 mg
Vitamin B6	.113 mg
Folacin	64.0 mcg
Vitamin 12	0
Pantothenic Acid (Vit. B5)	.471 mg
Vitamin E	21.0 mg
Biotin	19.0 mcg

Prominent Phytochemicals and Antioxidants in Almonds:
Vitamin E, Selenium, Essential Fatty Acids, Essential Amino Acids
Sources:
1) Santillo, Humbart, N.D. *Intuitive Eating.* Prescott, AZ: Hohm Press, 1993
2) *Nutrition Almanac*, Nutrition Research, Inc., McGraw-Hill, 1984. Nutritional data used with permission of the McGraw-Hill companies.
3) Margen, Sheldon, M.D. and the Editors of the University of California at Berkeley Wellness Newsletter. *The Wellness Encyclopedia of Food and Nutrition.* New York, NY: Rebus Press (Random House), 1992.
4) Blonz, Edward R., Ph.D. *The Really Simple No Nonsense Nutrition Guide.* Berkeley, CA: Conari Press, 1993. 1144 65th St., Suite B, Emeryville, CA 94608.

3

ALMONDS

WHAT IS SO GOOD ABOUT ALMONDS?

Protein

In the Kingdom of Proteins, Almonds are Queens! *Protein* is the word given to a collection of protein parts called *amino acids*. In the human body, dietary protein (from the foods we eat) is digested, or broken down into its component amino acids. These amino acids are then recombined through a variety of bodily processes into "human-use protein." Amino acids and human-use protein become major sources of building materials for all body tissues and a crucial ingredient for complex chemical processes such as hormone production.

There are approximately twenty-two amino acids that make up the primary components of complete human protein. Eight of these (some nutritionists/researchers are now saying nine, but we'll use eight to make this point and you'll get the picture) are called "essential amino acids" (EAA's). They are *essential* because although your body cannot manufacture them, they are necessary for building complete human protein. Therefore, you must get these EAA's regularly from the food you eat.

Luckily, you don't have to worry about ingesting all eight EAA's at the same time, since the body stores various components waiting for their proper companions to come along. When they're all in place, the body builds whatever it needs. However, it is a big plus when you *can* eat foods containing all the EAA's because then your body has a more certain supply of all the "makings" of the complete protein.

If a food does contain all the EAA's then it is called a complete protein. This is where almonds come in as the queens of protein. Almonds contain significant amounts of *all* of the essential amino acids in one delicious package!

Commonly we are educated to think that animal protein, such as meat or dairy products, are optimal sources of protein because they are complete protein foods, whereas most vegetables and fruits are incomplete protein. Notable exceptions in the plant kingdom are seeds such as almonds and sunflower seeds, and some beans, such as soybeans.

To get complete protein building blocks from incomplete protein sources, eat a wide variety of intelligently chosen foods, but don't forget that the protein you eat, whether animal or plant, must be digested into its component amino acids first. Only then will the amino acids be reconfigured into what your body needs.

In most instances, animal protein is harder to break down than plant protein. While the body is putting extra energy into the breakdown of animal protein, less energy and attention is available for other, often more rejuvenating processes that the body needs and wants to do—like resting an overworked digestive system, fighting an illness, or the continual repair and replacement of damaged or worn body tissues. Also, the byproducts of the digestion (or indigestion) of animal foods, such as the uric acid byproduct of meat digestion, contributes mightily to such conditions as arthritis. (I have never heard of anyone building up arthritis symptoms by eating too many vegetables!)

Scientists have verified that our over-consumption of animal products, including animal protein, causes grave negative side effects to our health. As mentioned in the Introduction, the Food Pyramid guide to a healthy diet (developed by the United States Department of Agriculture) bears this out emphatically, if indirectly, in recommending only 4 to 6 ounces of meat *or* 2 eggs as the *maximum* amounts of these foods per day. For many clever healthcare practitioners, even these "small" amounts are too high a recommendation for everyday consumption. Compare this moderate meat/dairy recommendation to the whooping 6 to 11 servings of grains *and* 3 to 5 servings of vegetables suggested per day on the Food Pyramid, and it is clear that the vegetable kingdom is undoubtedly our #1 resource for supplying the functional components needed for optimal health.

LALITHA RANTS:

For most of our lives we have been told to eat meat and dairy products, and plenty of them! "More protein, that's what we need!"

Next thing you know we are all suffering from nasty diseases such as arthritis, heart disease, kidney stones, high cholesterol ... and who knows what else! We are now learning that these illnesses are related back to all that meat and dairy.

I bet those meat and milk farmers had some "pull" in my old school district when my teachers were making me memorize the Four Food Groups which I just "shouldn't do without!" Meat and milk were lauded as if they were a major food group of their own, so most of the boys in my school equated their budding virility with eating a big steak and drinking a jug of milk as often as possible.

And where are these budding boys now? I'll tell you. Today they are the stiff, balding, heart-bypass victims, old before their time. The only healthy guys left are the "weirdo" vegetarians whose bananas we used to squash cruelly on the sidewalk.

Almost everybody today knows about the problems with this animal product consumption business, but so what! We're addicted, and besides, people ask, "Am I supposed to go against my entire childhood programming?"

What I'd really like to know is—why haven't all those studies about the unpleasant and slow deteriorization of health through eating animal products been put on the national news every day? Huh? Studies like the ones that fill great books like Jean Carper's Food Your Miracle Medicine, and Humbart Santillo's Intuitive Eating?

Well, now at least we've got the new Food Guide Pyramid, and "better late than never" as the unevolved, cliché-brained amongst us might say. (By the way, I never really smashed any "weirdo" vegetarian's banana; I just got carried away with my narrative.)

On the subject of animal protein versus plant protein, nutrition researcher Humbart Santillo, N.D., author of *Intuitive Eating* (see Recommended Bibliography) writes:

Many of you may still be under the impression that meat protein is the best. Experiments have proven that one can secure all the protein that is necessary from vegetable and fruit sources, and that the use of meat is both unnecessary and harmful. Meat also brings impure substances along with excessive protein into the body. Excess protein puts a stress on the digestive tract, kidneys, and liver and lowers the body's nerve energies.

Eating too much protein, especially animal protein (eggs, meat, cheese, etc.), places the body into a "luxuriant metabolism" where the catabolic (degenerative) processes of the body are stimulated. "Luxuriant metabolism" means the body is stimulated into a rapid burning off of the excess protein. This process gives us a sense of false strength. Uric acid, which is a byproduct of meat, metabolizes and acts as a stimulant (false strength), and is very irritating to the nervous system. In order to protect itself from excess uric acid, the body steals calcium, as a buffer, from the teeth and bones, and combines it with the uric acid to form calcium urate crystals, a less irritating substance, but one that can also lead to kidney stones, and rheumatic disorders. (p. 76)

Dr. Santillo is describing two health concerns here—first, our well-intentioned but ill-advised eating of *excess* animal proteins is over-stimulating us and giving a false sense of strength. Second, that same excess protein is also causing calcium to be depleted from other body tissues such as our bones. To top off the insult, Santillo claims that both of these factors are major contributors to premature aging!

Max Gerson, M.D., author of *A Cancer Therapy: Results of 50 Cases and the Cure of Advanced Cancer by Diet Therapy* (Barrytown, NY: Station Hill Press, 1990), along with the World Health Organization and Walter Willet, M.D. of the Harvard School of Public Health, all corroborate Santillo's statements in their own research. The consensus of these health professionals and others is that approximately 25 to 35 grams of protein in a day is plenty for an average adult (children may need more); and the preferred source of this protein is from vegetables. (See Chapter 13.)

You could easily get about 30 grams of protein in a single day from vegetable sources by eating one ounce of almonds and/or other seeds, such as sunflower or sesame seeds (approximately 5+ grams protein), and five servings of whole grain foods, like Brown Rice or legumes such as soybeans (approx. 25+ grams protein). Easy! Right? This reasonable amount is far from the recommended 60 or more grams of protein a day, preferably from animal products, which was the standard years ago. Prime sources of vegetable protein in the *10 Essential Foods* system are Almonds, Brown Rice (and other whole grains and legumes/dried beans), Sprouts such as alfalfa and bean Sprouts, as well as the Healthy Additions listed in each of these chapters.

If you are a non-vegetarian reading this, take heart. I am not a strict vegetarian either, because I regularly eat 2 or 3 ounces of fish, perhaps two times a week. For people who fit this "non-vegetarian" description, keep in mind that just 3 ounces of tuna packed in water gives a full 30 grams of protein by itself, before any of the rest of the day's foods are consumed. Therefore, it is wise to be educated and circumspect regarding amounts. (Read more about the long-term health effects of a high animal-protein diet in Chapter 13.)

For vegetarian protein, I love to eat my almonds after I have soaked them a few hours, or overnight, in water or pineapple juice. The almonds think they are being watered in preparation for making a new almond tree, and so they swell up. Then, their enzymes become activated and the germination process begins inside them. This means that the activated enzymes start pre-digesting all the components in the seed (almond), including the plant protein, for use in growing the new plant. When you pop them into your mouth for eating, presto!—predigested everything, including protein already broken down into amino acids ready for your use! This is such a wonderful trick to know that I suggest soaking not only your almonds but other seeds, such as sunflower or sesame seeds as well. You get much greater nutritional mileage this way. Especially for anyone who has poor digestion and gets gas or burps from eating any raw seeds such as the almonds, this soaking/predigesting trick is definitely the way to go. When any of my friends who need more vegetable protein complains of "finicky" digestion, perhaps because of pregnancy, illness or poor eating habits, I always recommend soaked almonds. *Voilà.* (See more information about sprouting in the Sprouts chapter.)

Attention Men!

Men who eat almonds receive a positive side-effect— almonds contain properties that enhance prostate gland health. This enhancement comes about through the particular richness of the alanine, glycine, and glutamic acid amino acids in almonds. The eating of seeds high in these amino acids has long been a folk remedy against enlargement of the prostate gland and the symptoms associated with it. Pumpkin seeds are the most famous for this quality, although almonds exhibit a similar amino acid content. Sesame seeds, flaxseed and saw palmetto fruit (a popular herb whose seed concentrate is sold in health food stores) are also good "prostate health" foods.

To use these foods for prostate health eat a total of one to two ounces a day of unsalted, raw or dry roasted pumpkin seeds, or a pumpkin seed and almond mixture, or a home-made seed "butter" made from a ground mixture of several of the seeds mentioned. (See the recipe under the KIDS LOVE THIS heading at the end of this chapter.) The world famous phytochemical researcher, Dr. James Duke of the USDA, has dubbed this type of mixture "Prosnut Butter."

"What About the Fat In Almonds?"

Yes, almonds contain fat. But it is a combination of several healthy types of fat that, in proper proportion to all else, will enhance your health.

I say "in proper proportion" because, for those of you who may tend to overdo a good thing, I suppose I should make it clear that I do not suggest eating lots of almonds everyday. One or two ounces (1-2 servings) within any given day is plenty, depending upon your calorie needs and your ability to digest the amount of almonds you are eating! In general, you would not depend upon almonds as your only source of protein and healthy fat. There are proteins in many other of the *10 Essential Foods*, Sprouted beans being one prime example; and for a rejuvenating dietary fat you should go for the Flax Oil.

Getting back to my point about the fat in almonds—without "healthy fat" our health would deteriorate miserably (see more about this in the Flax Oil chapter). For instance, one serving of almonds contain about 15 grams of fat, but only about 1.4 grams of the saturated type of fat we continually hear health warnings about. The other 13.6 grams is highly-usable, unsaturated fat.

Jean Carper, in her book *Food Your Miracle Medicine* (New York, NY: Harper Collins, 1993) reports:

> Dr. Gene Spiller had men and women with fairly high cholesterol, averaging 240, eat three and a half ounces of almonds a day for three to nine weeks. Others ate equal amounts of fat from cheese or olive oil. The average cholesterol of the almond eaters sank 10 to 15 percent compared to that of the cheese eaters. The almonds worked as well as olive oil [*for lowering cholesterol*]. This makes sense, says Dr. Spiller, because most of the fat in almonds and olive oil is chemically identical [*high in antioxidant monounsaturated fatty acids*]. (p. 52)

In his newsletter, *Health and Healing* (see Recommended Bibliography) of March 1995, Julian Whitaker, M.D., director of the Whitaker Wellness Institute in Newport Beach, CA. wrote about dietary fat intake and its unquestionable implication in many degenerative diseases. Whitaker asserts:

> I have learned since [*after his work at the world famous Pritikin clinic with Nathan Pritikin M.D.*] that the culprit is not fat but is primarily high intakes of animal fat, cholesterol, heated animal fats, heated vegetable oils, and excessive fat calories. Certain high-fat foods such as avocados, nuts and seeds are simply not a problem. We aren't a population ridden with heart disease and cancer because we eat too many avocados and walnuts; on the contrary, these food are important for achieving good health. (p. 7)

Boron

Almonds are a particularly good source of boron (as are fruits and nuts in general), along with Figs, Broccoli, Dulse and Spinach, four others of my *10 Essential Foods*. (See more about boron in the Dulse chapter.)

Few people had ever heard of boron, or known of its importance to health, until recently when boron made the news because of its implication in the treatment of osteoporosis.

Boron is a trace mineral, meaning it is found in the body in "trace" or minute amounts. For a long time boron was one of many trace nutrients that were thought to be of little importance to our health and belonged to that category of nutrients described by "role in human nutrition unknown." After all, how could a substance present in such minuscule amounts be all that important, right? As I will describe, its "secrets" are being uncovered.

In investigating the research on boron for this book, although almonds were often specifically mentioned in the "high in boron category", it was difficult to find nutritional-content data with an actual measurement of the boron in almonds. Just when I had given up hope on pinning down this detail, I spoke with Forrest Nielson, Ph.D., Center Director and Research Nutritionist at the USDA., Agricultural Research Service. He is one of the world's top experts in boron research. In speaking with him, he said it so happened that he had specifically mentioned the boron content of almonds in his article ,"Facts and Fallacies About Boron," (*Nutrition Today*, May/June 1992, p.6). Almonds was near the top of the list for boron content — 23 mcg of boron per gram of almonds. Therefore one serving of almonds, approximately 15 almonds (28 grams), would give you about .64 mg of boron — a very respectible amount when we are talking about a trace mineral!

However, I know that a food can only be high in boron (or many other minerals for that matter) *if the soil it is grown in can provide that boron*. (This is a very important point. The mineral content of soils and foods is discussed in more detail in the Dulse chapter.) When I asked Dr. Nielson about this, he said this was true to a certain extent, but that boron, for example, was an essential nutrient for plant growth and that any plant would not survive without at least some boron available to it, however small an amount. He explained that almonds were an example of a plant that needed higher levels of boron for maturation (as evidenced by the high boron concentration in the almonds) and it seemed reasonable that they might not even grow properly in boron-poor soils. Of course, a boron *rich* soil would likely produce almonds with the highest content of that mineral.

Over the last few years, the research of Dr. Nielsen is showing boron to be crucial not only in the absorption of calcium and magnesium, but, in post-menopausal women, boron's effect can boost estrogen and testosterone levels through reducing the loss of these hormones in the urine. These activities, amongst others, mean that boron is at least one actively important nutritional factor in the prevention and treatment of osteoporosis.

Without the presence of boron, simply taking a calcium supplement or eating "tons" of dairy products to help replace a lack of available calcium is not enough. As I just mentioned, it is now known that boron is crucial in the processes responsible for calcium's uptake into the body (along with magnesium which almonds are also rich in). In fact, if you are low on boron, you are more likely to be *losing* calcium no matter *how much* milk, dairy products and calcium supplements you are consuming! This is why most state-of-the-art calcium supplements now contain boron, among other synergistic ingredients, such as magnesium.

Boron is only needed in small amounts (3 mg. per day), and can easily be supplied from a daily intake of some combination of the boron-rich foods, including almonds.

Symptoms of a deficiency of boron, such as brittle bones, sluggish mental activity, and menopause symptoms, can often be helped by these dietary means. (Additionally, those with severe symptoms might take added boron in their calcium supplement, or alone, up to 3-6 mg. per day.)

Boron addresses mental sluggishness because of its affect on the electrical activity of the brain. Even though this is true of other trace minerals, boron is one that has been particularly researched in this regard. For instance, research psychologist James Penland, Ph.D. at the U.S. Department of Agriculture's Grand Forks Human Nutrition Research Center, found that when test subjects ate little boron their brain activity was notably more sluggish than when boron-rich foods were added back to their diets. In reporting this research, Jean Carper writes:

> When their diets [*the test subjects*] were very deficient in boron, their performance on the simplest tasks slowed down. They could not tap their fingers as fast, track a target as accurately with a computer joystick, or as rapidly pick out specific letters of the alphabet ... But when they went back on a high-boron regimen (3 milligrams a day) their brain wave activity picked up, as detected by electroencephalograms.
> From: *Food Your Miracle Medicine* (New York, NY: Harper Collins, 1993 p. 278.)

Unfortunately, agricultural practices in the United States and in the western world in general, tend to deplete boron from our soil and hence from our foods. Therefore, we have to be doubly conscientious in eating foods from the plant kingdom, especially those I mentioned, to give ourselves the best chances of getting boron as well as other nutrients. In my research I have often come across information showing organically grown foods to be higher in nutrition. This leads me to the hope that they might also be higher in boron. This line of thinking makes sense to me because the very principles of organic farming demand that organic farmers pay more attention to replenishing their soils in a thoroughly balanced fashion than do non-organic farmers. (In addition to a boron deficiency, a diet low in fresh foods and high in animal products and cooked or processed foods is typically one that leads to the premature aging and poor health commonly rooted in life-long nutrient deficiencies of *all* types.)

In case you are wondering, it would be very difficult to consume too much boron. You would have to get more than 50 mg. a day (impossible in a sane person's diet!) to even approach a boron "pig-out" which might result in an imbalance in other nutrients; but even then boron is considered non-toxic.

All in all, almonds are a concentrated and synergistic package of functional components including significant amounts of complete protein, along with calcium, magnesium, boron, vitamin E, and zinc—all of which enhance the health-promoting activities of each other.

Almonds, the Perfect Snack

Since almonds are also easy to carry around, they are an important snack food. Remember I am not talking about roasted, salted almonds here. Heating almonds causes the natural oils within them to begin deteriorating, i.e., to become rancid, at a rapid rate; and the salt is also a "no-no" for good health. If you must have roasted almonds, make them yourself in your oven at home. Roast them dry without added oil, little if any salt and eat them right away. I have a friend who, for special occasions, oven-roasts almonds mixed with a little Bragg's Liquid Aminos (a mildly salty soy-type condiment; see the Supplies Appendix B) and a few of her favorite spices. She bakes them at about 300 degrees for about 10 minutes or so. She stirs them two or three times while she is baking/roasting them, and then immediately serves them for a delicious treat.

For regular almond consumption however, the raw, lively ones are the best —the ones still able to sprout.

TASOLE: My student Jason had a wonderful knack for working with medicinal plants, and was a great comfort and support to the well-being of his friends—whenever he could stay awake that is.

"Jason, did you ever notice how you seem tired, unalert, or even sleepy at the most inconvenient times?" I asked. "For instance, every day for the last five days I see that you are trying to force yourself to keep alert even when you are involved in a project in which you have a genuine interest. Are you getting enough sleep?"

Jason gave me a discouraged look. "I get plenty of sleep, Lalitha, but I still feel a sudden drop in my energy every day, especially at mid-morning and late afternoon. I tried using those 'pep pills,' you know the ones I mean? I've tried the caffeine-type from the drug store, and the health store ones that stimulate with some kind of herbs, but they don't actually fix anything. I sure get pepped up for awhile, but then I crash worse than ever."

As I looked at him more closely I remarked, "That sounds just like low blood sugar. Have you had a health check-up lately?"

Well, actually I did," Jason spoke as he yawned. "I was told I had low blood sugar just like you said. Hypoglycemia, the doctor called it. She suggested I eat lots more protein, especially meat, but the more meat I eat the worse I feel. Then I get a craving for sugar, and soon I'm 'pigging out' on sugary snacks. I feel good for about an hour and then I'm in the pits again, feeling like I could just lie down and sleep all day. Something still seems out of balance and I guess I'll just have to put up with it. The doctor said it wasn't life threatening or anything."

"I used to be like that too," I told him, "until my healing teacher got hold of me. She saved my health in many ways. At the time I met her I had just passed a semester of school in which I drank shots of Tabasco Sauce between classes to keep awake all day. I couldn't handle caffeine, or I probably would have been drinking coffee. She taught me a great trick that brought me through a lot of bad days while I was doing more in-depth healing on myself under her guidance."

"A trick?" Jason questioned, as he perked up momentarily.

"Yes, a trick," I repeated. "Or rather a useful and actually healthy habit to practice."

It was getting to be early afternoon which was a time in the day that Jason was not at his best. I wasn't sure he wanted to hear about it right then but he answered somewhat grudgingly, "OK, tell me about it. But I've got to say that learning a new habit sounds like another piece of work to me. I feel tired just thinking about it."

"The basic idea is to attempt to keep your blood sugar as balanced as possible throughout the day so that you don't have those extreme ups and downs," I began. "There are many things that help with this and one of them involves eating raw almonds and raw honey in the right amounts and at the right times throughout the day. I use two empty 35mm film containers, those types with the tight-fitting snap-on lids, to carry honey and almonds around with me in my pocket, or in my book knapsack."

Jason objected, "That doesn't sound like very much food. I need to eat a lot."

"These are not gobble-down-all-you-want instructions," I replied. "I'm about to get to the part about amounts and timing, so listen up. This is the crucial part. When you are approaching a time of day when you know you often have an energy slump or sugar low, or maybe you are finding yourself already in the middle of the slump, stop for a minute and eat *one* almond. I literally mean one almond. Don't pop more than one into your mouth at a time. Chew that almond up really well before swallowing it. Pay attention to how it is tasting. If it tastes good and still 'almondy,' then put another almond into your mouth, chew it to a fine pulp, pay attention to the taste, and swallow. Usually somewhere in between one and six almonds you will notice the taste change. Some people describe it as chalky, or they simply say the almond looses its specific flavor and is beginning to taste a little blah. Right at this point when an almond changes flavor, go ahead and swallow that one but do not eat any more. Put the almond container away and get out the one holding the honey. Next, put a small finger-tip amount of honey into your mouth and notice how it tastes as it melts there before you swallow it. If it has an average amount of sweet taste to it, or less, then eat another finger-tip amount of honey. Notice how that next bit is tasting. Usually somewhere between one and six of these finger-tip amounts a person will notice the honey becoming sweeter in taste, maybe even sickeningly sweet all of a sudden, in some cases, and this is the signal to stop right then and eat no more honey. That's the basic scenario and you could do it several times a day. Let's give it a try right now," I offered as I finished this basic outline of the procedure.

"This sure doesn't sound like much of a snack to last me through the day," Jason stated skeptically as I got out my honey and almonds. "I don't see how it can help anything. But I like those foods, so, no harm in trying it I suppose."

That remark got me a little exasperated. "Jason," I said, "We are not talking about meal replacement here. I am trying to describe to you a way of balancing your protein-sugar level so that you will have more steady, long-burning fuel in your body throughout the day without the large ups and downs you find such a drag. Raw almonds are a good source of easy-to-digest protein, especially if they are chewed well; and raw honey is a good source of slower burning types of sugars (as opposed to the fast burn of the simple processed sugars in junk foods that give an energy high and then a big crash later). When you eat these two foods in the way I described, they help balance the protein and sugar needs of your body so that you have a better chance for steady energy without the crash. If you go crazy with throwing handfuls of almonds and honey into your mouth you'll go *way* past the point of balance without even noticing it, and I doubt if you'll feel that great. You'll probably get the same extreme ups and downs as before. But, this system of paying attention to the taste, one bite at a time, works very well, because when the flavor changes that means that your body chemistry has also changed."

While I was going through this further explanation, Jason was thoughtfully munching an almond. He actually completed the almond/honey procedure in a couple of minutes and by the time I had answered his questions he was already noticing some energy returning and the sleepy feeling definitely going away.

"I think I may have eaten an almond or two too many before I realized the flavor had changed," he said with a grin. "But I definitely feel better and I think I'll quickly get the hang of it. I'll carry this stuff around for a few days and give it a real try. Then I'll let you know how it works for me."

When I saw Jason a few days later he was smiling broadly. He had been doing "the almond and honey trick" (as he called it) two or three times each day, and it was working. I wasn't too surprised, as I had seen dramatic results for friends with more extreme low blood sugar problems. Of course, I thought it was a great idea when Jason told me he was going to start seeing a good naturopathic doctor to help him with more in-depth healing.

The Vitamin E Connection

Good dietary sources of the antioxidants vitamin E and selenium are almonds, Brown Rice and whole grains, Dulse and other sea vegetables, and Flax Oil, along with their Alternatives. Even though almonds are a good source of selenium, Brown Rice and Dulse have significantly more. (See more about selenium in the Brown Rice chapter.) You cannot expect to get the entire daily amount needed of these nutrients without especially including these groups (whole grains, nuts and seeds, sea vegetables and healthy oils) in your daily diet. Even with a diet rich in vitamin E foods, many health professionals still suggest a vitamin E supplement of at least 100 IU per day—that's how important they consider vitamin E to be. Vitamin E and selenium work closely together to promote elasticity of tissues (including arteries). Since they are antioxidants, these two substances help to slow the deterioration of body tissues and processes associated with aging and illness. Vitamin E plays a central role in the cellular respiration of all muscles, especially cardiac and skeletal; while selenium is also important in fertility and for the assimilation of proteins. Both are important in fat metabolism. These factors make vitamin E and selenium two of the "antioxidants of choice" for heart health, and many prominent studies support this.

Julian Whitaker M.D., in his newsletter *Health and Healing* of July 1993, cites a spectacular study of 87,245 nurses who took 100 IU of supplemental vitamin E for two years and ended up with 41% lower risk of heart disease than non-users of vitamin E! Author Jean Carper reports about Dr. Gary Fraser M.D. of Loma Linda University whose research on 31,208 participants led him to bluntly state that munching on a few nuts one to five times a week, perhaps an ounce or so "per munch," (and almonds were particularly mentioned among others) can, due to their vitamin E, high selenium, and mono-unsaturated fat content, be a preventive to heart disease.

The properties of vitamin E and selenium also make them important elements to strengthen our immune systems and lessen damage to our cells from all sorts of toxins and pollutants both internal and external.

It's All In the Zinc ... and Biotin

Are you interested in keeping your sex glands healthy, hormone production up to par, immunity in tip-top shape, and your brain functioning on all cylinders? Then you better be certain to get enough zinc in your diet, especially if you are a vegetarian. Good plant-based sources of zinc include: seeds, especially pumpkin seeds and almonds, and whole grains such as Brown Rice and whole wheat. Sea foods, especially shell fish, are potent zinc carriers from animal sources.

A final accolade to almonds is their biotin content. (Brown Rice are also good sources.) Biotin is a part of the vitamin B complex group. Since all the B vitamins are water soluble and excreted in the urine, they need to be replenished regularly. We either need to provide the raw materials for the body to synthesize them, (as it does for biotin,) or we need to ingest them in the diet. Although biotin is synthesized by intestinal bacteria in humans, it is still important to also have it in the diet. Biotin is needed for the metabolism and synthesis of fats, amino acids and carbohydrates—all major parts of the body's chemical processes!

SHOPPING FOR ALMONDS and OTHER FOOD SKILLS

From the moment seeds or nuts are shelled, their natural oils are exposed to light, air and perhaps extremes in temperatures. These environmental factors begin a deterioration process in the seed oils; at worst, the seeds can become fairly rancid. To some degree almonds are conveniently protected from the effects of these influences because they have that lovely brown skin still covering them after the shell is removed. Shelled sunflower seeds and other nuts and seeds are not so fortunate, however. You may be lucky, like I have been, in finding a store with a "cold room" where the consumer can dish up the bulk foods such as almonds and sunflower seeds from the bins kept there. But don't count on it!

Even though it is common to find these raw seeds in bags and bins, unrefrigerated and exposed to deteriorating influences, you can still make the best of a mediocre situation by keeping them under refrigeration when you get them home. Another shopper's trick is to shop at a store that has a high turnover in bulk goods. Buy smaller amounts more regularly so that you may get the freshest supply under the circumstances.

Don't hesitate to add whole, fresh, raw nuts and seeds such as almonds, sesame, and sunflower seeds to dishes you are cooking, or to salads and dressings you are preparing. They are great nutritional additions to the menu. My husband loves to eat his pasta with a small handful of almonds tossed over it. In my home, and in the homes of many of my friends, it is not uncommon to find ground, roasted sesame seeds or chopped almonds available in a small bowl as a wonderful condiment for sprinkling atop grain dishes, baked potatoes, steamed vegetables and salads.

HEALTHY ADDITIONS, ALTERNATIVES and TRAVELERS TIPS

Many other fresh nuts and seeds make fantastic Additions to almonds. In fact, it was an anxiety-producing experience to try to choose *one* to name this chapter after. Finally, because it is a complete protein and since I like the flavor of soaked almonds so much, I chose almonds.

You can apply much of what I said about almonds to many of these Additions, most notably sunflower seeds (higher in vitamin E than other nuts and seeds), pumpkin seeds (higher in zinc than other nuts and seeds), and sesame seeds. Brazil nuts are so rich in selenium that one cup can give you an entire day's worth of selenium (144 mcgs).

Even though peanuts have "good numbers" on nutrition charts, I don't recommend them (yes, contrary to some expert opinions), because I have observed their oils to be particularly quick to go rancid as soon as their shells are taken off. In my experience, peanut oil is hard on your liver, and hard to digest in any case. Also, growing underground as they do, peanuts are especially vulnerable to infestation of parasite eggs, most notably pinworms (and I have noticed a high incidence of pinworms in peanut-butter-fed children at daycare centers).

Fresh, uncontaminated fish can be a good choice as an Addition to the diet because of their protein and trace elements content. The key words here are "fresh" and "uncontaminated."

If you can detect any fishy odor in the so-called "fresh" fish you are inspecting for possible purchase, you can be sure it is not fresh at all, but in fact is starting to decompose. Unless you are certain of the purity of the waters from which the fish was caught, it is highly likely that the fish is full of health-destroying contaminants. Because of the severe marketing contaminations, environmental contamination and transportation contaminations in fish, unless you are catching your own in clean waters you must be circumspect in casually eating this once wonderful, but now often highly-contaminated protein food.

Water-packed canned tuna, especially if packed in this country, is a good choice. Also, as a protein sources for non-vegetarians, organic meats, poultry and eggs are better choices than the non-organic ones. (Read more about this in Chapter 13, on Meat, Fish, Poultry and Dairy.)

While traveling, or on a break from work, you can usually purchase nuts and seeds (perhaps walnuts, almonds, brazil nuts, or sunflower seeds) still in their shells in the produce department of a supermarket. This is the freshest and best. Just keep a nutcracker handy in your car's glove compartment and you are on your way! In bulk-food bins at many stores you can buy shelled nuts and seeds mixed with dried fruits, but beware of buying shelled nuts and seeds from open air markets in out-of-the-way places around the world. (Airborne contaminants, often present in dust-laden foods, are something to be wary of.)

Papaya John's Energy Bars (read all about them in the 10 Essential Snacks, Appendix C) contain ground almonds along with several other energy-producing ingredients. This is a go-anywhere way to get your almonds!

In restaurants, if I'm feeling like I need protein, I might go for the simple, unfried fish dishes. Or, I'm likely to look around for a good Mexican restaurant and get something with beans. At salad bars, I have occasionally seen shelled nuts or seeds.

SURVIVAL CHOICES for COMPROMISING CIRCUMSTANCES

Small packets of shelled, raw nuts and seeds can sometimes be found in the "baking goods" department of grocery stores. Also, most vending machines and convenience markets will carry dry-roasted nuts and seeds, either salted or un-salted. Either of these choices could make an OK snack, although these pre-packaged nuts and seeds have often been on the shelf and/or "in transit" so long that the oils they contain are often rancid (to varying degrees)—whether you can taste it yet or not. Your liver can probably handle a little of this; but don't overdo it.

KIDS LOVE THIS

In a blender, food processor, or coffee bean/nut grinder, grind fresh, raw almonds to a powder. (As an alternative you may want to grind a variety of seeds such as an almond, sunflower seed, sesame seed combination.) Grind enough to get one cup of powdered almonds, or whatever mix you like. To this seed/nut powder add one tablespoon of a healthy oil such as cold pressed Barlean's Flaxseed oil, sesame, sunflower, or almond oil, and two tablespoons of pure water. Continue to add one part healthy oil to two parts pure water until you get a consistency somewhat like sticky clay. You can add a dollop of honey to this mixture if you like.

Next, mold this sticky mixture into seed balls of a size to your liking. Roll these balls in a mixture of shredded coconut and roasted carob powder (a light brown, sweet and tasty powder of the carob bean available at health food stores). Keep refrigerated. Serve these nut-seed balls as a high-protein, high calorie, high-energy snack for active people, especially children. For higher calorie content use more oil and perhaps less water.

STEAMED GARLIC BROCCOLI

3/4 cup broccoli flowerettes
1/4 cup sliced broccoli stems
3/4 cup sliced leak (the white part and the tender green part)
1 clove garlic, minced

Steam the broccoli stems. When slightly soft, add the flowerettes, the leek and the minced garlic. Steam until slightly soft.

Suggested Additions: Melted butter or olive oil and/or lemon juice and/or soy sauce.

FUNCTIONAL COMPONENTS
In 100 Grams Fresh, Raw Broccoli
Serving Size: 1/2 cup (50 grams) raw broccoli

Calories	28.0
Protein	2.98 g
Fat	.35 g
Carbohydrates	5.24 g
Fiber	1.11 g
Cholesterol	0
Calcium	44.0 mg
Phosphorus	66.0 mg
Magnesium	25.0 mg
Potassium	325.0 mg
Sodium	27.0 mg
Iron	.88 mg
Copper	.045 mg
Manganese	.229 mg
Zinc	.40 mg
Selenium	*yes
Chromium	**11.0 mcg
Vitamin A	1,900.0 mg
Vitamin C	93.2 mg
Vitamin B1 (Thiamin)	.065 mg
Vitamin B2 (Riboflavin)	.119 mg
Vitamin B3 (Niacin)	.638 mg
Vitamin B6	.2 mg
Folacin	71.0 mcg
Vitamin 12	0
Pantothenic Acid (Vit. B5)	.535 mg
Vitamin E	0
Biotin	0

Prominent Phytochemicals and Antioxidants in Broccoli:
Carotinoids (vitamin A), vitamin C, zinc, indoles, chlorophyll, phytosterols, sulforaphane, selenium, lutein.

Sources:
1) Santillo, Humbart, N.D. *Intuitive Eating* (Prescott, AZ: Hohm Press, 1993).
2) *Harvard Health Letter* April 1995, p.10.
3) **Carper, Jean. *Food Your Miracle Medicine* (New York, NY: Harper Collins, 1993).
4) Margen, Sheldon, M.D. and the Editors of the University of California at Berkeley "Wellness Newsletter." *The Wellness Encyclopedia of Food and Nutrition* (New York, NY: Rebus Press [Random House], 1992).

Recipe From: Nostrand, Carol. *Junk Food to Real Food* (New Caanan, CT: Keats Publishing, 1994, p. 218.) Used with permission.

4

BROCCOLI

WHAT IS SO GOOD ABOUT BROCCOLI?

Broccoli is a spectacular vegetable. Besides being easy to grow-on-your-own, it is fabulous for preventing disease and building health. Broccoli is a member of the cabbage family called *cruciferous*. Other examples of the cruciferous family are red and green cabbage, kale, chard, cauliflower, mustard greens, rutabaga, turnip, and radish. Actually, all of these cruciferous vegetables are stand-outs for many of the same reasons as broccoli, so anything I write about broccoli can also be applied, with a little flexibility, to these other vegetables.

Cruciferous vegetables are available all over the world in one form or another. I picked broccoli to shine in this chapter partly because it is one of my personal favorites in this group, but also because it is well researched and has been extolled for its health benefits in popular magazines, such as *McCall's* (Dec. '94) and *Newsweek* (April '94), which certainly has added to consumer interest in this brilliant blast of vitality we call *broccoli*.

All the Fuss About Indoles

Indoles are a phytochemical group. Broccoli contains high amounts of indoles, perhaps more than any other vegetable. Indoles have now been identified as a cancer-preventive that works in a very specific and clever way. Since carcinogens must be activated by hooking onto a particular enzyme in the body, certain indoles race over to those same enzymes and hook up in the "parking spot" before the carcinogens can get there. This action blocks the carcinogens from getting activated. Without the proper "parking spots" or hook-ups within our body's chemistry, carcinogens are not able to damage the body's cells. As a primary example, specific indoles are known to neutralize and help get rid of the type of estrogen which can promote breast cancer.

Because of indoles and other functional components in broccoli, there is no doubt of its top-of-the-list status as a disease preventing food. Phyllis and James Balch (C.N.C. and M.D. respectively), in their book *Prescription for Cooking* (Greenfield, IN: PAB Books Publishing, 1987), report that eating broccoli "lowers the risk of cancer, primarily cancer of the colon, esophagus, larynx, lung, prostrate, oral cavity, pharynx, and stomach."

One little catch is that, to get the greatest good out of the cruciferous indoles, one must eat them raw or lightly cooked. Heavy cooking tends to destroy them.

TASOLE: Each summer my friend Tina and I like to take a short trip to a river not too far from our town. We don't want to use up too much of our sitting-around time fussing with a lot of food preparation, or food storage, yet at the same time we don't want to pig-out on quick-fix junk foods. If we do get around to cooking anything it is usually for one meal a day, and this one meal gets simpler year by year. In this way we give our digestive systems a rest and a gentle clean-out by eating fresh fruits and vegetables, and drinking lots of pure water most of the day. However, it did take us a few years to finally narrow things down to the perfect camping diet for our particular style and taste buds.

"The main thing I want to do for the next few days is just sit by this river and read," I told Tina as we drove nearer to the dirt track that led in towards the brush along the river bank.

"Me too," Tina agreed. "We'll eat when we get hungry and only cook if we feel like it. Let's stop at that grocery store just before the river turn-off and see what we feel like bringing to eat."

"Right," I said, as I turned into the parking lot of the grocery store.

We parked near the front door, anticipating a big haul of goodies and a quick dash out of there, wanting no time wasted. Once in the store, however, it was a bit of a different story. This was our first day out and we were still experiencing the "regular life buzz" as we called it. That's when the "grocery store zombie mode" began to get us. We were hooked! Hypnotized by the packaging and seemingly unlimited choices, we pushed our cart over to the so-called *Healthy Snacks* department.

"Let's get some of this granola," Tina suggested.

"Sure, but then how about some liquid to get it wet?" I responded

"Do we need to get it wet?" Tina wondered out loud. "OK. Just in case, let's get a jar of pineapple juice. Not canned juice, though; too junky," she answered herself.

I put my head around the next aisle and got excited. "Chips! Let's get chips. Then let's go to the bulk aisle for some trail mix."

"If we get chips, we'll need some salsa," Tina reminded me. "And let's get some dried fruit while we're here in the bulk aisle. Yogurt, do we need yogurt?"

"What about cheese and crackers?" Tina added brightly.

"Mustard for the crackers, then," I said.

Our shopping cart filled as we sleep-walked around the store, forgetting the simple idea we had in mind upon entering. Soon we drifted into the produce department.

"Lettuce looks good; and tomatoes; we'll want some sort of salad dressing, eh? "

"We could cook up some of these onions with potatoes, what do you think?," we bantered back and forth as we put anything we liked into our cart (which was getting quite full, to put it mildly).

For the most part our choices were good ones, but ... Then, like an alarm clock rousing us from a dream we spied a table piled high with ... fresh broccoli!

"This is exactly what I feel like eating. Piles of broccoli!" Tina was more enthusiastic than ever.

"Me too," I said. "Look how fresh it is, how green and crisp; and what a great price!" (Broccoli really gets us going. We're serious broccoli fans!) Reaching for the choicest bunches, we remembered our purpose.

"Hey, wait a minute. What are we doing!" Tina laughed as we turned to each other with our armloads of broccoli and no room for it in the shopping cart.

"Look at all this stuff!" she gasped. "We've got sauces, dressings, delicate lettuces and milk products. They all need to be refrigerated; that means ice and trips to the store for more ice and a bigger cooler. We'll be chopping onions and potatoes for the larger cooking pan we don't have yet; and then think of the clean-up! We'll make efforts to eat all this stuff even if we don't feel like it because we won't want it to spoil before the ice melts. What happened to the simple, no fuss plan we started out with?"

I looked at our overloaded cart and had to admit that there were also things in there that we normally wouldn't even buy—like the pretend hot dogs made from texturized vegetable protein (TVP) filled with all sorts of who-knows-what to make the mega-processed mess palatable. In silent agreement, and with a sigh of relief, we immediately started retracing our steps to put most of the items back on the shelves. Starting over, we returned to the broccoli pile.

The following day at the river we began to settle into the true sit-around mood we had come for. And, each of our remaining four days went on like this. We would wake up to a beautiful dawn and eat a Grapefruit (one of the other *10 Essentials*, don't forget) or orange, or grab a piece of raw broccoli to munch on (sometimes dipped in salsa). Next, we'd float on the river ... or sit in it ... or sit next to it in our chairs, while reading, sleeping, chatting or day-dreaming. All the while, we had regular access to the chilled herbal sun-tea in our one small ice chest (which also held more broccoli), the citrus fruit, and salsa for the chips we did not put back during the grocery store escapade. On an energetic day we often steamed a large amount of broccoli for lunch, and we always steamed an extra large batch of broccoli for every dinner, without fail. In addition to the broccoli at dinner, we would cook up a pot of our favorite whole grain—buckwheat. We had some olive oil and Bragg's Liquid Aminos (a salty-flavored, soy-based condiment; see the Supplies Appendix B) to add to the steamed broccoli, or buckwheat, if we felt like it. Broccoli raw; broccoli steamed for lunch; broccoli steamed for dinner with buckwheat—broccoli was the main event!

Every evening we faced our chairs towards the sunset waiting for our buckwheat to cook in the one pot we had. Our chairs were close enough to the cooking pot, set on our one-burner propane-powered stove, that we didn't even have to get up from our sunset-watching to lift the pot lid and check on it. When the buckwheat was cooked, we divided it into our two bowls, added the Bragg's and olive oil, and began eating it as an appetizer while we piled broccoli into the pot for the main course. Often two pots of steamed broccoli were called for before the dinner was considered properly accomplished. Both Tina and I felt wonderfully satisfied. Just our river-sitting style!

Even though much of the research involving phytochemicals—such as those in broccoli—cites the lessening of cancer activity as a prominent issue, the lessening of *all disease activity* is more to the point in my opinion. As you know, the health of your immune system is the bottom-line of defense against disease, whatever it is. Well, guess what? Hundreds of phytochemicals, including the indoles I've just described, support the immune system in a colorful variety of ways which are so numerous that we can't even guess at them all (although I am sure that researchers will keep trying). And, I have found that anything which enhances the action of the immune system to help prevent such drastic diseases as cancer, also helps against the more "common" types of inconveniences that plague our health—such as chronic infections, fatigue and allergies.

"Sulpho ... What?"

Sulforaphane, another phytochemical found in extraordinary concentrations in broccoli, is active in cancer and disease prevention in animals. Reporting in *Newsweek*, April 1995, Sharon Begley in her article "Beyond Vitamins," about phytochemicals, stated that sulforaphane quite dramatically kept lab animals from getting breast cancer. Furthermore, when researchers at Johns Hopkins Medical Institution added sulforaphane to human cells *in vitro*, it boosted the synthesis of anticancer enzymes. I too am convinced of sulforaphane's important role in disease prevention in humans. We need more non-rat research. Don't you agree?

Antioxidants Unlimited

Broccoli is a strong source of so many antioxidants that I will only be able to mention a few of them here; hopefully enough to whet your appetite for the vast possibilities of this wonder-vegetable. Beta carotene (vitamin A), vitamin C, selenium, zinc, lutein, folic acid and phytosterols are among the antioxidants in broccoli. Some of these antioxidants are discussed more extensively in other chapters (see: Almonds, Spinach, Brown Rice and Carrots). For instance, while broccoli has a generous amount of beta carotene, Carrots have still more; and Spinach boasts a higher content of lutein and folacin. Selenium is present in cruciferous vegetables, but more quantities are found in whole grains like Brown Rice, or in sea vegetables like Dulse.

These powerful antioxidants protect against damage to our cells from all sorts of attacking substances, including tobacco smoke, allergens, pollution, pathogens and carcinogens. Phytosterols, found in broccoli and all cruciferous vegetables, compete with dietary cholesterol for uptake in our intestines. The intestines pick up the phytosterols which then block the uptake of unhealthy types of cholesterol. Blocking unhealthy cholesterol limits the risk of heart disease. (See more about phytosterols in the Brown Rice chapter.) A healthy serving of broccoli several times a week, or other cruciferous vegetables, covers a lot of bases!

The Minerals in Broccoli

Broccoli is an excellent source of certain minerals and trace minerals. Chromium, for example, a blood-sugar balancer almost without equal, is a prominent trace mineral in broccoli. In my own experience I have found chromium to be highly useful for both low and high blood sugar problems. Jean Carper substantiates this balancing of high or low blood sugar, in *Food Your Miracle Medicine* (New York, NY: Harper Collins, 1993, p. 422), where she specifically mentions chromium's value in treating diabetes, low-blood sugar (hypoglycemia), and in lessening the need for insulin and/or medications. She quotes Richard A. Anderson, Ph.D., at the USDA's Human Nutrition Research Center in Beltsville, MD as saying: "Whatever the blood sugar problem, chromium tends to normalize it."

Dr. Anderson is one of many doctors, scientists and health researchers who cite an almost epidemic deficit of chromium in the human population. This deficit contributes significantly to all types of blood sugar problems. When the depleted chromium is replenished in the body, however, the blood sugar problems often lessen or disappear altogether. Personally, I have witnessed this many times.

About 90% of Americans are chromium deficient, an unquestionable indication of the mineral depletion in our soils as well as our poor dietary habits. Broccoli, especially organically grown, can supply us with a hefty daily dose of this vital mineral. One cup of broccoli could provide as much as 22 mcg. of chromium out of the approximately 200 mcg. needed as a healthy maintenance amount (according to some researchers). Dulse, other sea vegetables, barley and other whole grains, and nuts are also good sources of chromium, although broccoli tops the list.

Dr. Michael Colgan of the Colgan Institute of Nutritional Science in San Diego, CA suggests that the general chromium deficit is so profound that we need to aim for amounts along the lines of 200 to 800 mcg. per day. He suggests the highest amounts for athletes, but I have seen these 800 mcg. amounts work miracles for blood-sugar-challenged folks from all walks of life.

Chromium from foods is the most potent, in my opinion; so eat chromium-rich foods as much as you want. In addition to broccoli, outstanding sources of chromium are found in whole grains (especially whole wheat), apples, corn, cucumbers, onions, prunes, mushrooms and dry beans. Also, almost all of the 10 Essential Foods have significant amounts of chromium, especially if organically grown. In his book Intuitive Eating, Humbart Santillo includes a Chromium Chart which allows you to easily figure out how to get more of this desired nutrient. You learn, for instance, that one medium apple gives you a whopping 36 mcgs.! One cup of broccoli gives 22 mcgs. of chromium.

In addition to trace minerals such as chromium and selenium, broccoli supplies usable amounts of major minerals, including calcium, phosphorus, magnesium and potassium. (Figs are higher in some of these major minerals and Dulse has more of the trace minerals, but hey, we can't be eating Figs and Dulse all day long as our only source of these indispensable items, can we?) These minerals are present in all vegetables to varying degrees. Eating foods like broccoli, which are high in these major minerals, is proven to keep blood pressure at a healthy low, protect against stroke, build strong bones, soothe nerves, and in general keep all of the complex cellular chemistry working optimally for peak health.

One cup of broccoli gives you: calcium 88 mgs., phosphorus 132 mgs., magnesium 50 mgs. and potassium 650 mgs. When you consider that anyone who gets an extra 400 mgs. of potassium a day lessens his or her chances of a stroke by 40%, eating a cup of broccoli, or other cruciferous vegetables, several times a week is certainly a tasty insurance policy. (Yes, I do believe "insurance" is an ideally appropriate word when applied to the subject of fresh whole foods and their role in helping you maintain optimal health!)

SHOPPING FOR BROCCOLI and OTHER FOOD SKILLS:

If you pick up a stalk of broccoli at the grocery store only to find that it will bend back and forth like rubber in your hands, don't buy it. The broccoli you want is bright green overall (or green with a purple flowering top, in the case of purple broccoli), with dense flower tops that are not yellowing, and stems so crisp they would snap off if bent; and slender stems if possible. Slender (and therefore tender) stalks are a big plus in the "broccoli hunt" when you can find them. But this may not be the usual case; at least it isn't at the stores in my town.

LALITHA RANTS:

Broccoli is a powerhouse of functional components, and don't those produce guys (or gals) know this? Don't they know that we shoppers know this too?

I wonder, what are they trying to do, those produce people, with their whimpy, wobbly broccoli, with stalks so thick they've got to be the tough old ancestors of the fresh tender stuff that the gourmet cooks are probably getting!

What about us regular cooks, huh? If we won't buy this rubbery stuff does that mean we don't get any at all? Can't convince me that the soft broccoli with the yellow tinges is some special hybrid ... and supposed to be that way. Phewy! It's loosing its phytochemicals, that's what it's doing!

What? What was that they told you? That it doesn't matter that much?

Well, it matters to me!

That yellowish, rubbery broccoli may get peddled to somebody so that grocery store profits won't go down, but its not fooling me for a minute. If I simply wanted wilted plant fiber, and didn't care about taste, phytochemicals and nutritional quality, well ... er ... I might as well eat my neighbors new brush pile!

And another thing! I know about that trick they do of tying the broccoli together so the stalks hold each other up, so I always check in the middle of those clumps for spoilage, and I give those tied-together broccoli stalks the same gentle bending-test I give to the loose ones!

Thicker, tougher stems denote more advanced age. And, while there are high concentrations of nutrients in the stems of broccoli (often higher even than in the flowering tops), if you have to peel a tough skin off of an older stalk of broccoli to be able to eat it, then you are also peeling much of these nutrients off as well. Perhaps this sorry situation is just one of those broccoli traumas we simply have to live with.

Oftentimes, broccoli comes with some leaves still attached, but if we don't know better we pull them off and throw them away. These leaves are highly edible and, like the tender stalks, can contain higher amounts of nutrients than the flower tops that get the most culinary attention. So, eat the leaves in soups, chopped in salads, or as part of a batch of steamed greens you may be preparing anyway.

If you are one of those cooks who wonders where the bright green color goes when you cook broccoli, I will solve the mystery for you right now. *You are overcooking it.* Please stop doing this. Overcooking ruins many of broccoli's best qualities—chlorophyll for one, the phytochemical that makes the broccoli green. The object of cooking broccoli is to do it lightly and quickly, without drowning it in water, or boiling it in oil. Your aim is to end up with a bright green color and a texture crispy yet just tender enough to bite through. Steaming or light stir-frying is perfect for this.

Don't underestimate the power of raw, fresh, tender, young broccoli tops with slender stems. When dipped in a delicious sauce, raw broccoli is pleasing to diners young and old alike. Many prefer it to the cooked varieties! While lightly-cooked broccoli provides significant nutrition to any meal, the highest concentrations of functional components are found in the raw broccoli.

If you are a person who says that any cabbage-family vegetable, including broccoli, is a little difficult for you to digest, seems to cause gas, or just doesn't smell good to you, there are a couple of things to try before giving up on these nutritional gold mines. The problem might simply be that you are overcooking your broccoli. The *Wellness Encyclopedia of Food and Nutrition* (by the editors of the University of California at Berkeley "Wellness Newsletter," New York, NY: Rebus Press, 1992, p.67) explains that:

> Heating broccoli (or any cruciferous vegetable) causes chemicals in the vegetable to break down and release various strong-smelling sulfur

compounds, including ammonia and hydrogen sulfide (the culprit behind the smell of rotten eggs). As broccoli cooks, more of these compounds are released, intensifying (rather than weakening) the odors. Some of the compounds also interact with chlorophyll, gradually turning the broccoli brownish the longer it cooks. As a result, it is best to cook broccoli rapidly in a small amount of water to minimize these chemical interactions [*and also to maximize the retention of nutrients*].

Some of the compounds released in cooking can also contribute to indigestion. Many people find that one form of broccoli (either the raw or the cooked) is easily digested while the other form is not. I've found no consistency in reports for one side or the other, but it is worth experimenting with both raw and cooked broccoli (and other cruciferous vegetables). Try both forms and determine which works best for you.

Another option for the indigestion-prone is to accompany broccoli-eating with taking a digestive enzyme (available at most health food stores) particularly suited for digesting beans. (I like *Beano*, a liquid enzyme suited for this purpose. Another brand, Prevail, produces a *Bean & Vege Enzyme Formula* in a tasteless powder in capsules.) Beans and cabbage-type vegetables undergo many of the same chemical interactions with cooking. Therefore, digestive help comes from the same direction. If you are just beginning to add more whole foods to your diet, these tricks will allow you to extract and use the fullest nutrition from all types of foods. After using whole foods regularly, your body will probably get so healthy and its digestive capacity so greatly enhanced, that digestive enzymes may be needed only on special occasions.

HEALTHY ADDITIONS, ALTERNATIVES and TRAVELERS TIPS

Any member of the cruciferous (cabbage) family of vegetables makes a good Alternative to broccoli; examples include kale, cabbage, cauliflower and chard. For Additions, choose any fresh vegetables you happen to like, especially those in season in your area.

Those who want the health benefits of living foods, but find that their lifestyle makes this difficult, have the choice of buying a high-tech "live food" supplement. Two of the best I have found are:

1) *Phyt-Aloe*—a primarily organic, raw, flash-dried, whole foods concentrate which contains the phytochemical and nutritional equivalent of eight ounces of fresh-squeezed plant juice (in one capsule) from nine different vegetables (including broccoli), and from three different fruits. This power-packed product retains over 90% of the phytochemicals and over 80% of all the vitamins, minerals, plant digestive enzymes and soluble fiber from the source fruits and vegetables. Besides *Phyt-Aloe*, the capsule version, there is a chewable version called *Phyto-Bears* for children and adults. These taste so great that children will fight you for more! Sold by Rejenitec Company. (Mail-order, see Supplies Appendix B.)

2) Whole leaf *Wheat Grass* and *Barley Grass* in tablet form; organic, raw, and flash dried, which gives the consumer a nutritionally significant dose of chlorophyll along with the functional components from these potent foods. Produced by Pines International, Inc. (This and several other excellent "green food supplements" are available at most health food stores. See Green Foods in Supplies Appendix B.)

Frozen broccoli still retains good nutrition and can be used when fresh is not available. Properly dehydrated vegetables including broccoli, especially if organic, are an excellent addition to fresh vegetables in the diet. They are a potent yet light-weight food for hikers and other travelers.

For travelers in general, some type of cabbage-family plant is grown almost everywhere in the world. If you find yourself in a part of the world where broccoli is not commonly grown, simply browse through the open-air market until you spy a vegetable that reminds you of any member of the cabbage-family. Such a vegetable might be reminiscent of kale, cauliflower, cabbages of all types, bok choy or Swiss chard, etc. Finding a locally grown substitute for broccoli will seriously support your good health on the road.

SURVIVAL CHOICE for COMPROMISING CIRCUMSTANCES

Frozen dinners containing "fresh" broccoli would be a good choice for quick preparation. Avoid canned broccoli and other canned vegetables if possible, because the canning process is so rough on nutrients. However, canned broccoli is not totally lacking in redeeming qualities; so, no reason to starve yourself if canned broccoli is the only choice available.

Since broccoli is so readily available, almost any restaurant will have it on hand for use in salads, soups, or as the vegetable *du jour*. Although not often listed separately on a menu, most restaurants have it available in their kitchens and are happy to send it forth freshly steamed, if you ask politely.

KIDS LOVE THIS

Many food preparers are surprised to find out that children often like raw broccoli better than cooked—especially when the broccoli is fresh and young.

Make a tasty dip, surround it with small broccoli flowers and watch it all disappear. Live-culture plain yogurt mixed with a little honey is a delicious dip that children gobble up. (Don't make the mistake of putting more than a dab of honey in the yogurt, however; and don't make the broccoli chunks too big.) Bite size pieces are usually the most popular.

Steamed broccoli is often well-liked by children, especially if it is served simply and not mixed with lots of other vegetables. Give your kids a chance!

One more recipe I have to pass along:

CURRIED TOFU AND BROCCOLI

1 small head broccoli
1-2 Tbs. olive oil
1 1/2 cups chopped mushrooms
1/2 pound firm tofu, cut into cubes
1 small can tomato juice (about 6 oz.)
1 1/2 Tbs. curry powder
2 tsp. cumin

Cut the broccoli into bite-sized pieces. (Peel the stalk and slice it, and cut the top into small flowerettes.)

In a large fry pan, saute the mushrooms in olive oil till lightly brown. Add all other ingredients except the broccoli. Simmer on a very low heat, covered, stirring occasionally, for about 1 hour.   (If there isn't time for the long, slow heating, just cook it until the tofu has absorbed the flavors.)

Add the broccoli and simmer another 1/2 hour. (Here again, to quicken cook-time if you need to [and to heighten nutrition], steam the broccoli for 10 minutes, then add it to the fry pan.)

Serve over rice. Non-fat plain yogurt is good as a condiment.

Recipe from: © Carol Anne Nostrand Johns, June 1996. Previously unpublished; used with permission.

PILAF CASSEROLE (serves 3 to 4)

1 Tbs. olive oil
3 Tbs. chopped onion
(about 1 small onion)
1/2 cup chopped mushrooms
(2-3 large mushrooms)
1 cup uncooked grain—brown rice, bulghur, buckwheat, millet or a mixture of them
2 Tbs. chopped green pepper
1 Tbs. chopped parsley
1/2 cup chopped celery
1 small carrot chopped
2 cups vegetable stock and 1 Tbs. soy sauce or use miso broth
Optional: add 1 tsp. sage or cumin
Preheat the oven to 350°

Heat the oil in a 1 quart casserole. Lightly saute the onion, mushrooms, and grain, then add the stock and any spices. The amount of broth depends on the type of grain used in the recipe. [For brown rice, use 1 cup brown rice with 2 cups water or broth. I have also found this to be approximately true for almost any grain combination.] Bring the liquid just to the boil, stir, cover and reduce the heat to the lowest possible temperature. Gently simmer 15 minutes. Add the vegetables, put the casserole in the oven and bake, covered, at 350° for 30 to 40 minutes, or until all the liquid is absorbed and the grain is "dry," yet tender. Note that this casserole is not meant to hold together particularly well. Rather, it is a light and fluffy mixture of grain and vegetables.

FUNCTIONAL COMPONENTS

In 200 Grams Cooked Brown Rice
Serving size*: 1 cup cooked brown rice, approx. 200 grams
(*Note: While the USDA Food Guide Pyramid considers 1/2 cup cooked rice to be a serving, I will use one cup cooked brown rice to equal one serving unless otherwise noted in my text.)

Calories	222.0
Protein	6.0 g
Fat	1.8 g
Carbohydrates	46.0 g
Fiber	.68 g
Cholesterol	0
Calcium	20.0 mg
Phosphorus	166.0 mg
Magnesium	86.0 mg
Potassium	86.0 mg
Sodium	2.3 mg
Iron	.84 mg
Copper	.2 mg
Manganese	2.0 mg
Zinc	1.26 mg
Selenium	25.73 mcg
Chromium	4.5 mcg
Vitamin A	0
Vitamin C	0
Vitamin B1 (Thiamin)	.19 mg
Vitamin B2 (Riboflavin)	.05 mg
Vitamin B3 (Niacin)	4.0 mg
Vitamin B6	.29 mg
Folacin	8.0 mcg.
Vitamin B12	0
Pantothenic Acid (Vit. B5)	.57 mg
Vitamin E	1.0 IU
Biotin	6.0 mcg

Prominent Phytochemicals and Antioxidants in Brown Rice:
Vitamin E, zinc, selenium, phytosterols, folacin, lignans.

Sources:
1) Santillo, Humbart, N.D. *Intuitive Eating* (Prescott, AZ: Hohm Press, 1993).
2) Margen, Sheldon, M.D. and the Editors of the University of California at Berkeley "Wellness Newsletter" *The Wellness Encyclopedia of Food and Nutrition* (New York, NY: Rebus Press (Random House), 1992).

Recipe from: Nostrand, Carol. *Junk Food to Real Food* (New Caanan, CT: Keats Publishing, 1994, p.231.) Used with permission.

5

BROWN RICE

WHAT IS BROWN RICE?

I used to think there was only one type of brown rice—healthy, but generally uninteresting. Brown rice was brown rice was brown rice, and that was it! When I was thinking this way, I realize now, I must have been just a cut above being brain dead. Over the years since then I have become a brown-rice-eating-fool ... with no end of creative choices in sight!

There are four major parts to a kernel of rice: the rough and inedible outer hull, which is always removed for human consumption; the bran; the germ (reproductive embryo); and finally, the starchy inner core. These last three parts comprise the majority of the kernel and contain its outstanding nutritional characteristics. How these parts are handled should be important to us as consumers. Based on what is done to them, the rice is referred to as "brown," "parboiled,' "precooked," or "converted white."

All rice is not equal! Brown rice is the least processed, and for our purposes as one of the *10 Essential Foods*, brown rice describes any rice that still has the bran and germ of the grain in place. Brown rice is not pre-processed or heavily milled, as is the case with parboiled or precooked (types of processing), or white rice (rice that has been heavily milled). With the bran and germ in place covering the inner kernel, the brown rice still retains a majority of its functional components for optimal nutritional content (i.e., vitamins, minerals, phytochemicals, fiber, etc.). It also renders a rich variety of flavors, textures, aromas and colors. This is especially true if the brown rice has been left growing to its complete maturity before harvest, thus allowing for the full development of functional components such as phytochemicals. One of the major brown rice producers in the United States (and one of my personal favorites), Lundberg Family Farms in Richvale, California, practices this optimal harvesting method for crops intended for brown rice milling, although this is not true of all rice producers.

WHAT'S SO GOOD ABOUT BROWN RICE?

Phytosterols, Etc.

Brown rice has approximately 9% to 12% protein and is full of many nutrients including trace minerals, B vitamins, iron, zinc, thiamin, niacin, calcium, phosphorus, potassium, magnesium and folacin. The bran layers of brown rice and other whole grains include a highly-unsaturated oil—rich in vitamin E and phytosterols (plant sterols, a type of phytochemical)— which, along with the significant fiber content of the rice, can contribute markedly to lowering the bad types of cholesterol, and can relieve and/or help prevent constipation and bowel disease.

Marcia Zimmerman, M.Ed., C.N. (in "Nutrition Science News," *Natural Foods Merchandiser,* September, 1995) reported on phytochemicals and phytosterols. After pointing out that phytosterols occur in most plant species, with green and yellow vegetables having significant amounts, Zimmerman explained that most of the research on this class of phytochemicals has been done on yams, soy, rice, herbs and pumpkin seeds.

> Phytosterols compete with dietary cholesterol for uptake in the intestines. They have demonstrated the ability to block the uptake of cholesterol (to which they are structurally related) and facilitate its excretion from the body. Cholesterol has long been implicated as a significant risk factor in cardiovascular disease ... Other investigations have revealed that phytosterols block the development of tumors in colon, breast and prostate glands. The mechanisms by which this occurs are not well understood, but we do know that phytosterols appear to alter cell membrane transfer in tumor growth and reduce inflammation.

Within the bran layers of whole grains like brown rice are plant lignans, known for their help in building immunity and preventing disease (see Flax Oil chapter). Whole grains also contain useful amounts of folacin (folic acid), a B vitamin. While Spinach is the highest in folacin of most vegetables, brown rice and whole grains are notable as well. Scientific literature shows that Folacin helps prevent birth defects (especially when given as a supplement), builds healthy blood, and is important for the reproduction of healthy cells. It is also vital to the use of protein; necessary for optimal liver performance; and invaluable protection against cervical, lung and pancreatic cancers.

Selenium Reigns!

Brown rice and other whole grains are a superb choice as a source of the antioxidant mineral selenium. (Dulse is at the top of the selenium-content list, and Almonds also have some to offer). Since I have already discussed this important mineral in the Almond chapter I will repeat only a few of the basic facts here to reinforce the case.

The benefits of selenium mentioned here are reaped by having at least 100 to 200 micrograms a day—directly from food or as a supplement. Some reputable nutritionists suggest twice that amount. At the moment there is data possibly indicating that selenium may be toxic when consumed in amounts of 750-1000 mcgs. a day over an extended period of time. This amount, however, would be very hard to exceed using only dietary sources—unless you ate six or seven cups of Brazil nuts, for instance, every day for an extended period of time (one cup of Brazil nuts can give you as much as 144 mcg's). That's a lot of nuts! Also, when you intake selenium from dietary (food) sources rather than supplement tablets, you are also ingesting other minerals and nutrients which work synergistically with the selenium, balancing it and making it, I believe, less likely to ever cause a problem. Until more definitive research is done, however, experts suggest staying within this 100-200 mcg. amount.

You can get 25 mcgs. of selenium in one serving of brown rice. Eat a few Almonds and other servings of various whole grains and you are easily up to the 100-200 mcg. mark.

Selenium is a great mood elevator. A deficiency of selenium can be accompanied by symptoms of anxiety, depression, mental sluggishness and fatigue. As a dynamic antioxidant, selenium helps prevent damage to body tissues caused by stress, pollution of all sorts, inflammation and high cholesterol. Selenium is one of four antioxidants (vitamins E, C and beta carotene are the other three) now touted as a primary combination for boosting the immune system while lowering chances for disease, including cancer and other tumor growth. Selenium is important in heart health since it improves the elasticity of arteries.

A Fantastic Fuel

The complex carbohydrates (starch) and naturally-occurring sugar content of brown rice are delightfully easy to digest and are prime sources of fuel. These complex carbohydrates provide a stable release of energy over a long period of time. Therefore, the blood sugar remains more consistently stable and one doesn't feel hungry so quickly after eating a main course of brown rice or other whole grains. This feeling of satisfaction (of having plenty of fuel to burn, and a more balanced blood sugar) after a good brown rice meal can diminish cravings and encourage us to eat less often.

The United States Department of Agriculture recommends using its newly developed Food Guide Pyramid for determining the amounts and types of foods to eat for optimal health and longevity. (See Figure 1.1.)

The Food Pyramid confirms what a majority of world cultures have always known. Namely, that grains such as brown rice form the center and foundation of a healthy diet. (Unless your circumstance is like that of the Eskimo culture, which has a diet high in animal meat and whose climate often prevents the growing of grain!) In fact, in Japan the word for *meal* is the same as the word for rice: *gohan*.

The USDA suggests six to eleven servings of foods from grains each day, and 1/2 cup of cooked brown rice, for example, is what they consider as one serving. (In my Functional Components list at the beginning of this chapter I consider 1 cup cooked brown rice as one serving. This would be equal to two USDA servings.) I strongly suggest that you eat only *whole grain* products for these servings. Of course, in order to carry out both the USDA's and my recommendations, you will want to become familiar with a variety of whole grains (see the Healthy Additions and Alternatives listed below) and the numerous forms they come in. At the same time, make it a point to keep your focus on my first choice in this category—brown rice of all types.

TASOLE: On a "smell-good" spring afternoon I heard the telephone ringing insistently and finally decided to answer. (I
guessed it was a friend who knows my frustration with a
frequently ringing phone, and my response of not answer-
ing every time.)

"Lalitha," the voice on the other end was almost frantic.
"He won't eat anything but brown rice. I'm not exaggerating! Bowls of brown rice with a little *Bragg's* sprinkled on
it. [*Bragg's* is a condiment with similarities to soy sauce.] He
doesn't even want sweets, and I know he gets plenty of
that at his mom's."

I immediately recognized the caller as my neighbor John
who I knew must be talking about his six-year-old son
Michael. Michael had just arrived for his three-week visit,
and John and I were about to have a "divorced-father-on-
his-own-with-young-son" conversation, similar to talks
we'd had over the past few years.

"How many days has he been home with you so far?" I
asked.

"He's on his third day. His mother doesn't like to hear a
report from Michael that all he is eating is brown rice, and
I guess it makes me nervous too," John admitted.

"We've talked about this before, remember?" I assured
him. "Brown rice is an extremely nutritious food. In fact, I
know several adults who don't hesitate to eat solely brown
rice for a few days, or even a few weeks at a time, as a healing and balancing regime whenever digestion or general
metabolism is upset from long-term traveling, poor eating
habits, or whatever. Michael usually starts off his visits this
way, so what's the big deal?"

"You're right. Michael does this every visit. The longest
he has ever gone has been six days before he willingly
begins adding more variety to his diet. I don't want to force
other foods on him because I've learned that just makes
him feel self-conscious and unhappy around food in general." John was regaining composure.

"Does he seem to be healthy in all other ways?" I wondered out loud. "For instance, does he have good energy?
And how is his general mood?"

John responded thoughtfully. "At first he seemed to
have that lethargy and moodiness which his mother says is
characteristic, and which I often see upon his arrival. I've
got to say, though, he certainly gets energetic after about

the second day of eating these brown-rice-only meals. Now that I think about it, his moodiness is greatly lessened also. Is that normal? I mean, is it OK to let him insist on eating only brown rice for days on end? Maybe I should take him to the doctor."

I tried to be tactful in what I brought up next. "I know Michael's mom is wonderful and watches Michael's health carefully, but their diet *is* quite heavy on sugar, meat and processed foods," I reminded John. "Such a diet is commonly known to encourage sluggishness. Michael seems to be intuitively trying to correct for this when he visits you. Of course, there is also the psychological stress of visiting between parents. His body simply knows what it needs to rebalance; then he is off and running. It doesn't sound to me like a doctor's visit is called for."

"And he always does begin asking for other foods after a few days," John added, comforting himself.

"What does he ask for?" I asked curiously. Inwardly I had a quick, uneasy fantasy of a child who switched from requests for brown rice to demands for only cakes and candies. (My fantasy child sat on a bed of cotton candy. A flying fire truck circled his bed and sprayed any desired sweet out of its fire hose and into his mouth on each go-around!)

"After days of eating only brown rice it is always the same pattern," John explained. "First he adds the carrot sticks, and then the celery sticks, along with his brown rice. Then he branches out into pasta, an occasional sweet, some fruit, some chicken—quite a variety now that I think about it. I guess I just like hearing you say its OK every time this happens."

"It doesn't sound to me like you have much to complain about!" I laughed. "I have many friends who are still wondering when their children will ask for a vegetable. Your own diet habits have had a good influence on Michael, I think. Feel free to call me later," I offered, as John said good-bye.

I saw John and Michael several times during the following three weeks of Michael's visit, but we didn't get a chance to talk much. A week or so after that I saw John without Michael.

"What happened this time? How long did the brown rice diet last?" I was curious.

"Six days," John shook his head and smiled. "I thought he was going for a record, but then he took a carrot stick out of the salad bowl at dinner. Of course, he still had some brown rice each day, but by the end of his visit Michael even tried some of my famous Caesar salad—and that was a welcome surprise!"

SHOPPING FOR BROWN RICE

I get new eye-openers about simple foods every day. One of my latest discoveries is that a shopper has to be careful even when buying a product in a bag that is blatantly labeled *Brown Rice*. While traveling together recently, a friend bought a bag of brown rice and brought it back to the house where we were staying. When she started measuring it into the pot I became a bit suspicious. As a seasoned connoisseur of brown rice I thought the rice didn't look quite right. My friend gave me the look that said, "Lalitha, don't be such a fanatic! It says *brown rice* and it is just regular brown rice. Quit being so paranoid!"

I couldn't stop myself from looking more closely, however. The kernels were somewhat rough, with a beige tinge, and looked like steamed rice kernels that had split open a little and then been dried. (You had to know what you were looking for to notice it, though.) I knew that whole-grain, unprocessed brown rice comes in many colors, from creamy white (not the stark white of milled white rice) to black. But unprocessed rice is smooth, not rough; and the kernels are not split open as the present ones were. Then I read the package more carefully. In the tiniest print were the words "parboiled brown rice'" Ahah! I was right!

"Parboiled" means rice has been steamed before milling. (This is different than precooked rice, and is sometimes referred to as "converted rice.") To be completely fair, parboiling is not the worst thing that can happen to brown rice as, during the process, a small amount of the water-soluble nutrients are forced into the inner kernel and saved; therefore, parboiled brown rice is on my Survival Choice list at the end of this chapter— for when you simply can't do better. At least with parboiled brown rice the consumer still has rice fiber left.

More commonly, however, after the parboil process, the rice is then milled into a white rice. Parboiling is a process for mainly cutting down the consumer's cooking time, insuring that the grains will remain fluffy after cooking. In any case, as you surely know by now, it is *not* my first choice. I want all the nutrition and flavor that the various brown rice have to offer left intact to be released when I prepare it.

LALITHA RANTS:

Parboiled! Steamed ahead of time! That does it. Can't even trust the darn labels on anything without reading all the fine print. It takes a person half a day and a dictionary just to get plain unprocessed rice—unpolished, unsteamed, unboiled, unsprayed, un-anythinged.

Parboiled of all things! Most parboiled rice is polished to a nub and then stored for who knows how long. And if you want a real bowel-clogger just try eating that type of white rice regularly—like a lot of Americans do!

And "enriched" rice? Do food manufacturers think we have white rice for brains, or what!? You can never enrich rice back to what it was. There are components that cannot be replaced synthetically, I don't care what they say. Even if a person goes for the "enriched" white rice, the so-called "enrichment" washes off or gets thrown out with the extra cooking water through uninformed cooking methods.

It washes off! Can you believe it?!

Well, there's not much to be said for leaving it on either, but ... Bad word #@! Bad word! Bad word!*

Precooked rice is just that—rice that has been cooked and then dehydrated and packaged. The cooking process commonly involves using large amounts of water that is then thrown away. Since many of the nutrients in rice are water-soluble, a great deal of nutrition literally goes down the drain. In addition, if the precooked rice is white rice, which it usually is, well ... I'll restrain myself from ranting again this time. The main advantage to precooking is that it produces a product that makes the consumer's preparation time quite short.

White rice is rice that has usually been harvested before fullest maturity, as this makes for a more efficient milling process. White rice has been milled (polished) until the hull, bran, and germ of the rice have been completely removed, thereby destroying the major sources of functional components (including fiber and nutrition), along with much flavor, color and texture. White rice leaves the consumer with a fairly bland, nutrient-low and, to me, quite useless product which many producers then "enrich" with a few synthetic nutrients to make it OK with us that they took all the good stuff out.

Milling is the primary difference between brown and white rice. This means that you and every other consumer will have a choice between, for example, brown Basmati or white Basmati (different millings of a specific type of rice loved by many rice connoisseurs), or the generic brown or white rice (different millings of the most commonly available and usually less expensive type of rice). Next, you have to determine (by careful inquiries and/or package-reading) if the rice being considered has been "parboiled," "precooked," or "enriched," and whether or not this is what you intend to buy.

The Spice of Life

The wide varieties of rice from around the world—each with a unique flavor and aroma—include many different types of brown rice. I regularly eat: long and short grain traditional brown; sweet brown rice; Wehani; Black Japonica; California Basmati; Indian Basmati; Texmati; and Wild Rice. (Wild rice, by the way, is technically not a grain, but is actually a grass seed. Wild rice is higher than brown rice in protein and B vitamins, as well as other nutrients; is more expensive, and is often mixed in with brown rice to create wonderful cuisine.)

The most affordable brown rice is the traditional long or short grain, commonly labeled generically as "long-grain brown rice" or "short-grain brown rice." These two are found at most food stores. The less familiarly named brown rice types, such as Wehani, Japonica, or Basmati, are commonly available at health food stores and gourmet food shops. I buy the generic brown rice, either short or long grain, for my staple rice. Then I mix in about 1/8 to 1/4 part (by dry measurement) of one of the other types and cook them together. This way I end up with a great variety of flavors and colors in my rice while still staying within my budget. Keep in mind that the color of a food relates to its phytochemical content. So, my mixtures not only give different nuances of nutritional content but different influences of phytochemicals (whose names usually remain unknown to me).

Did you know that brown rice is made into rice cakes (a round, cracker-like food that is generally served with a spread of some sort), rice milk (a good alternative to ordinary milk), rice milk frozen dessert (made from sweet brown rice and quite delicious), and Amazake, to name just a few? (Amazake is a thick, creamy, somewhat sweet, nutrient and protein-rich drink made from a rice base and possibly flavored with other ingredients such as Almonds or fruit. It has a consistency reminiscent of thick cream.) All these rice creations are available at health food stores; while some, like brown rice cakes, are available at most supermarkets too.

Rice is so versatile that it can be the main course for almost any eating opportunity. Rice cereal for breakfast with cinnamon and honey! An aromatic mixture of rice with vegetables for lunch or dinner. Or, as a snack, how about rice cakes spread with Almond butter or fruit conserves? Yumm ... Writing about food sure gets my appetite going.

Have Rice, Will Travel

Brown rice is a great traveling food. I have a fold up, one-burner propane stove that is so compact it can fit in the glove compartment of my car, or in a travel bag. I also have a two-cup stainless steel cooking pot, with a lid that also doubles as my eating dish. If I know I'm going to be on the road a lot, and subjected to restaurant food frequently, I don't hesitate to cook a half cup of rice in my hotel room whenever I want a nutritional energy boost. If I have any guests in the room when the rice is being cooked they usually cannot resist the delicious aroma, and ask for a taste. After one mouthful they almost always want more. Now I plan ahead by cooking a cup or more if I know someone is likely to appear at "snack time." To accompany the rice I always carry (or buy on the road) small bottles of olive oil and *Bragg's* (a salty-flavored liquid soy condiment), and I'm all set. Another perfect accompaniment to brown rice is Dulse. In addition to compatibility of flavor, aroma, and food-group types, Dulse adds trace minerals and vitamin B-12, which the brown rice lacks.

COOKING GREAT RICE and OTHER FOOD SKILLS

For cooking brown rice, here is a general plan to follow. Keep in mind that 1/2 cup uncooked brown rice yields about 1 1/2 cups of cooked rice.

General Rice-Cooking Plan

1. Start with a good pot—that means a pot that will adequately hold the amount of rice you want to cook, realizing that every 1/2 cup of dry rice will triple in size when cooked (1/2 cup dry rice

will equal 1 1/2 cups cooked rice), and you will be adding water to an amount double the amount of dry rice you start with. My idea of a good pot is stainless steel, if possible. (I never use an aluminum cooking pot because there is just too much evidence that toxic forms of aluminum in the diet [easily put there through cooking with aluminum implements] contribute to serious health problems. See more about this in chapter 2 under Guideline 6.)

2. Measure the desired quantity of rice and water into the pot. For each one cup of dry rice, add two cups of water. Usually 1/2 cup dry rice per person is a good amount to estimate and, if cooking for large quantities (more than two cups), lessen amount of water to 1 1/2 cups water to 1 cup rice. By the way, rice, since it always has its inedible outer hull removed, is very clean and does not need to be washed before putting it in the pot for cooking. In fact, washing can destroy delicate oils on the surface of the rice grains; and in the case of "enriched" rice, washing can actually wash off the so-called enrichment!

3. With a lid on the pot, bring the rice/water mixture to a boil. When it starts to boil, turn down the heat to a "very low simmer" and simmer approximately 45 to 60 minutes. (On my electric stove, I start out on "high" temperature to get the rice to a boil, and then immediately turn it all the way down to between "warm" and "low" heat.) Once the rice is brought to a boil, it will steam itself to "doneness," if kept on this very low heat *with the lid left undisturbed.* In other words, don't keep lifting the lid to check on the rice until at least 45 minutes have passed. You will soon get the timing perfect—based on the amounts used, type of pot, electric or gas stove, etc.—and then you'll never have to lift the lid until the rice is done. The rice should be thoroughly cooked. A good test for this is to pinch a grain of rice between your thumb and ring finger and the grain should easily mash

totally flat with no stiffness or sensation of grittyness.

4. If your rice turns out cooked, yet too soggy, you
    have used too much water. If it feels crumbly or
    gritty, it has not cooked long enough, or there
    was too little water in the pot to finish the cook-
    ing process. In general, look for a thoroughly
    cooked, yet light and fluffy consistency.

Many rice connoisseurs use different pots, timings and mea-
surements than what I am suggesting. Try my way and if it
doesn't suit you, experiment with your own changes. Rice can
be cooked in other liquids besides water—vegetable broth, or
diluted tomato juice (1/2 water to 1/2 juice) work well, for
instance. Even though electric rice cookers are now available,
all the ones I've found have some aluminum parts which come
in contact with the boiling water or the rice itself. Beware! For
me, a ceramic, electric "crock pot" serves when I can't be
around to watch the pot.

HEALTHY ADDITIONS, ALTERNATIVES and TRAVELERS TIPS

Good Alternatives to brown rice are any other edible,
unprocessed whole grains including but not limited to: millet,
buckwheat, quinoa, amaranth, barley, rye, wheat and corn.

Like rice, some of these Alternatives have the same tough,
inedible outer hulls or seed coverings which need to be partly
milled or "pearled" away. Generally, however, the grain will
not be totally polished off down to its central core, as is the case
with white rice. Barley and buckwheat are examples of such
partly milled grains. Therefore, lightly "pearled" barley is OK
in the *10 Essential Foods* scheme, as is buckwheat which will be
found with its inedible outer shell milled off. (This will generally be called *whole buckwheat groats*.) Still, there are differences
in how grains such as barley and buckwheat are
processed/milled. A discerning shopper will develop an educated eye. If I want pearled barley, for instance, I look for barley which still has a brownish-beige tinge to it, indicating that
some of the bran covering is still in place. The grain is not totally pearled down to its white and shiny core. The same is true
for hulls of buckwheat. Even after the tough black outer seed
hull of buckwheat is removed, the buckwheat grain/seed still

has a lovely tan-colored inner skin (bran and germ) that contributes to its extraordinary protein content and its great flavor. As tasty and nutritious Additions, I highly recommend all types of dried beans/legumes such as: anazazi beans, adzuki beans, pinto beans, lentils (both green/brown and red), split peas, corn, soy beans and black turtle beans. (Surely someone in my reading audience is already objecting that beans are not in the same category as grains as far as the USDA Food Pyramid goes. This is true, but the USDA doesn't run my life and many of us know that the "mood" of beans and rice is so similar as to link them together profoundly, at least in the philosophical sense.)

Beans are higher in protein than many grains (notable exceptions in grains are quinoa, buckwheat and amaranth which have more protein than most beans). And, while beans have functional components in common with the grains (as well as the "mood" I mentioned), this protein content is probably why beans are listed more near the top of the Food Pyramid along with the other protein foods (recommended at 2-3 servings per day instead of the 6-7 servings per day suggested for the grains). This 2-3 serving per day amount is smart when it comes to protein foods, such as milk, red meats, fish, nuts, etc. However, I don't agree at all when it comes to the dry beans. So, I'm putting them in as an excellent Addition in my brown rice/whole grain group, declaring that you can eat them as much as you like. (Unless the amount you like is turning you into a chubby little nugget, or a gaseous ball of noxious fumes ... I'm sure you know what I mean.)

First choice for travelers could be some of the delicious brown rice "meals-in-a-box" from Lundberg Farms. I often take along a one-burner propane, or an electric one-burner hot-plate when I travel so I can whip up a rice meal in my hotel room or at my camp site. If you are careful about where you eat, a savvy traveler can get some good fast-food beans inexpensively while on the road. However, you have to ask the right question (*Is there lard in your beans?*) when buying ready-to-go beans, unless you want to end up with a serving of beans which was just an excuse for selling you a plate of lard.

If traveling in a country where rice is a staple, plain rice or "rice-from-the-pot" can be a tasty treat (this rice is less likely to have been refried in rancid fats or oils). In a country where beans are a more common staple, in Mexico for example, try "beans-from-the-pot" (*frijoles de la ollo*). I have asked for these at many a small café or restaurant and it has been a great choice.

Just as with the rice, these beans directly from the cooking pot of a food-seller are often less likely to have yet been cooked in lard or other rancid fats or oils as they are not yet "refried."

SURVIVAL CHOICES for COMPROMISING CIRCUMSTANCES

In this general category of grains and beans, try to get the least processed products you can find which still appeal to your taste buds. These survival choices could include, but are not limited to: parboiled whole grains; frozen TV dinners centered around whole grains or beans (yes! there is such a thing, but you'll probably have to search out a health food store to find them); prepackaged quick-cook rice mixes (the Lundberg Farms brand is quite good and even has a quick-cook rice cereal for breakfast); plain canned beans without lard; and steamed white rice (try to avoid fried rice) at a restaurant if eating out.

KIDS LOVE THIS

Use leftover, cooked brown rice as a breakfast cereal. Grind up the cooked rice in a blender with a little water to make your desired consistency. Heat it up and serve the smooth warmed cereal in a bowl with a dab of butter or a spoonful of Flaxseed Oil; add honey and cinnamon (to taste) and serve.

Some "customers" like a small amount of milk on their cereal, but this is not necessary. Alternatives to cow's milk are soy or rice milk, which are available in a variety of flavors (children often prefer the vanilla-flavored ones) at health food stores and many grocery stores.

Lundberg Farms makes a boxed, quick-cook rice cereal that some find convenient. If the breakfast cook has the time, raw rice can be ground up in the blender to make your own rice cereal from scratch. In a sauce pan, put the ground rice and three times the amount of water as ground rice. Simmer for approximately 20 minutes or less, until there is no grittyness left in the cereal.

Another recipe not to miss:

WILD RICE 'N PASTA
1/4 cup cooked wild rice
1/4 cup cooked Jerusalem artichoke spaghetti
6 almonds, chopped
1/4 cup soft tofu
1-2 Tbs. sliced celery
2 Tbs. chopped parsley
2 Tbs. sliced green leek
1 Tbs. butter/olive oil combination
2 tsp. soy sauce

Lightly sauté the almonds and leeks in the butter in a fry pan. Add all other ingredients and stir until warm. Add the soy sauce last, to taste.

This serves one person with a good appetite. Increase the amounts for serving more than one.

Recipe from: Nostrand, Carol. *Junk Food to Real Food* (New Caanan, CT: Keats Publishing, 1994, p.232). Used with permission.

CARROT SALAD

4 cups grated carrots (about 4 medium carrots)
1/2 cup chopped walnuts
1/2 cup soaked currants or raisins
1 cup diced apples and/or pineapple
2 Tbs. shredded coconut
Optional: 1/2 cup sunflower seeds

Mix and decorate with sprigs of parsley. Top with Honey Dressing.

HONEY DRESSING (makes 1/3 cup)

Combine and shake well before using:
1/2 cup sunflower or sesame oil
2 Tbs. honey
1/4 tsp. lemon juice

FUNCTIONAL COMPONENTS

In 100 Grams Raw Carrot
Serving Size: 1/2 cup raw carrots, 55 grams (approximately 1 medium carrot)

Calories	43.0
Protein	1.03 g
Fat	.09 g
Carbohydrates	10.14 g
Fiber	1.04 g
Cholesterol	0
Calcium	31.0 mg
Phosphorus	30.0 mg
Magnesium	13.0 mg
Potassium	227.0 mg
Sodium	66.0 mg
Iron	.62 mg
Copper	.134 mg
Manganese	.752 mg
Zinc	.30 mg
Selenium	1.65 mcg
Chromium	5. mcg
Vitamin A	
(from Beta Carotene)	28,129.0 IU
Vitamin C	2.3 mg
Vitamin B1 (Thiamin)	.034 mg
Vitamin B2 (Riboflavin)	.056 mg
Vitamin B3 (Niacin)	.506 mg
Vitamin B6	.246 mg
Folacin	13.9 mcg
Vitamin B12	0
Pantothenic Acid	
(Vitamin B5)	.304 mg
Vitamin E	yes
Biotin	2.25 mcg

Prominent Phytochemicals and Antioxidants in Carrots:
Beta carotene (17 mg.) calcium pectate, vitamin C, selenium.

Sources:
1) Santillo, Humbart, N.D. *Intuitive Eating* (Prescott, AZ: Hohm Press, 1993).
2) Margen, Sheldon, M.D. and the Editors of the University of California at Berkeley "Wellness Newsletter," *The Wellness Encyclopedia of Food and Nutrition* (New York, NY: Rebus Press [Random House], 1992).

Recipes from: Nostrand, Carol. *Junk Food to Real Food* (New Caanan, CT: Keats Publishing, 1994, pp.

6

CARROTS

WHAT IS SO GOOD ABOUT CARROTS?

Carrots are amazing—and versatile too. As a young "apprentice healer," I drank carrot juice everyday. Then, in the next moment, my teacher would show us how to use the carrot pulp (right from the juicer) as a poultice for healing the burned skin on a neighbor's hand. (The neighbor had popped in, needing immediate help with a burn from cooking.)

Let me give you an overall list of "What Carrots Can Do For You," taken from *Prescription for Cooking* by Phyllis A Balch, C.N.C. and James F. Balch, M.D. (see Recommended Bibliography).

Carrot

- Powerful antioxidant
- Builds healthy skin and tissue
- Good for heart disease
- Reduces risk of cancer (especially lung)
- Helps stop diarrhea
- Stimulates appetite
- Helps build healthy teeth
- Improves eyesight
- Prevents eye and mucus membrane infection
- Aids diuresis
- Aids in recovery from illness, especially as a juice

As I continue discussing the functional components which are responsible for these health-enhancing attributes, don't be surprised if you start craving a big glass of carrot juice!

Beta Carotene

Carrot lovers (or *wanna-be* carrot lovers) unite! Don't settle for wimpy, light-orange carrots once you know that the darker the orange color of your carrots, the more beta carotene is present. Why should you care about this little fact?

Because beta carotene strengthens the action of our all-important immune system, and this in turn results in the enhanced ability to fight off ordinary colds and flu as well as such potential "killers" as cancer, stroke and heart disease.

Beta carotene is proven highly useful in healing the body's irritated mucous membranes in those suffering from allergies, ulcers, colds, diarrhea, or sore throats. It positively enhances glandular balance and liver function, which easily deteriorates in many of us due to drinking alcohol, smoking cigarettes, and the stress and pollution of daily life. Anyone with eye weakness, eye strain, nerve deterioration or night blindness should take note that the beta carotene in carrots, and in other fruits and vegetables, can catalyze the much-needed help for these strained eye nerves and other eye tissues.

Do you have scaly or dry skin? Beta carotene could be a missing link.

One of my purposes in *10 Essential Foods* is to emphasize the importance of getting vitally-alive functional components/optimal nutrition in the whole foods that we eat. However, many of the components I mention are also available as food supplement tablets, and beta carotene is at the top of this list for many people.

There has been some controversy associated with beta carotene, however. In 1995 the Beta Carotene and Retinol Efficacy Trial (or CARET study) was halted because the researchers found possible adverse effects in the subjects. The news media had quite a field day with this. In this study, large doses of synthetic beta carotene *and* vitamin A (50,000 IU of beta carotene and 25,000 IU of vitamin A) were given each day to half of a group of 18,314 high-risk-of-cancer participants (heavy smokers or people who had prolonged exposure to asbestos).

The CARET study indicated that the supplements (the vitamin A and beta carotene) actually contributed to a *higher* rate of cancer in the test subjects. However, many rebuttals have articulated the faults of this study. Julian Whitaker, M.D., author, practicing physician, and director of the Whitaker Wellness Institute in Newport Beach, CA, in his newsletter *Health and Healing* (March 1996, p.5), wrote about loopholes in the CARET study, while reiterating to his readers the importance of maintaining beta carotene in their diets and as a daily supplement.

> First, large doses of synthetic beta carotene and vitamin A were given in isolation. Fresh fruits and vegetables [including carrots] contain hundreds of carotenoids, of which beta carotene is just one. In addition, these particular antioxidants were given without any additional supplemental antioxidants. Natural food contains a broad spectrum of nutrients in balance, and you should strive for this same balance in your nutritional supplementation program. We know that all nutrients work synergistically, and that taking large doses of single nutrients can cause serious imbalances in your body, even illness. That's why ... I emphasize taking a full spectrum of nutritional supplements in addition to a balanced diet that includes abundant fresh fruits and vegetables for optimal health.
>
> Second, the subjects in this study were among those at the highest risk for getting cancer ... This is not a normal population. The purpose of nutritional supplementation, especially of the antioxidant group, is the prevention of chronic disease in the general population.

In the *Wellness Letter* of the University of California at Berkeley (July 1996, p.7) experts were asked about the safety of taking a multi-vitamin supplement containing what the questioner described as "5,000 IU's" of beta carotene. The answer to this question addresses the confusion about the relationship between vitamin A and beta carotene, as well as the safety of beta carotene in whole foods such as carrots.

> Such a multivitamin is safe. First of all, that's not much beta carotene, which is usually measured in milligrams. The IU's (international units) listed on vitamin bottles refer to *the*

> *amount of vitamin A the beta carotene could be con-*
> *verted to in the body.* 5000 IU's is the RDA for vit-
> amin A for men, which is the amount supplied
> by 3 milligrams of beta carotene. A medium-
> sized carrot provides about 12 milligrams.
>   Second, it is far from definite that beta
> carotene pills pose any danger, and *there is*
> *absolutely no evidence that beta carotene in foods is*
> *dangerous.*

Vitamin A, itself, is a fat-soluble substance found in animal
products such as fish and eggs. Not being water soluble, it is
not excreted in the urine and remains in the body until it is
used up or broken down. Because it can be stored, vitamin A
can be toxic to the liver in amounts starting at 25,000 IU's a day
when ingested over a sustained period of time. Beta carotene,
however, is a phytochemical found in plants. The body uses
beta carotene to make vitamin A on an "as needed" basis. Beta
carotene is non-toxic. When beta carotene is available in the
body but there is no present need for it to be made into vitamin A, it is available to perform other functions as an antioxidant.

Jean Carper, a health researcher and author of *Food Your*
Miracle Medicine (see Recommended Bibliography), sat next to
me while we were both signing books at a national health trade
show recently. This is where I first became aware of her
astounding research work. In this particular book Jean cites
studies from all over the world which validate the amazing
healing and health-promoting significance of beta carotene.
While I am not going to repeat all the research data here, I will
share a few juicy highlights.

One Harvard study showed that women who ate one large
carrot every day cut their risk of heart attack by 22 percent.
Another Harvard study, involving 90,000 nurses tracked for 8
years showed that eating carrots 5 times a week or more could
cut a nurse's risk of stroke by a welcome 68 percent! Ms. Carper
states that in nearly all the studies she has reviewed in the past
ten years, the most enthusiastic beta carotene eaters [Carrots,
Spinach, Broccoli and pink Grapefruit rating high as source
foods] were "only 40 to 70 percent as likely to get lung cancer"
as those who had low levels of beta carotene in their diets.
Researchers at the University of Alabama have shown that
women who eat carrots (also other high beta carotene foods
such as Spinach or Broccoli) at least once a day, have 27 percent

less chance of getting cervical cancer as those who eat those foods less often. The "list" of beta carotene examples for enhanced immune action and therefore better health is quite long, to put it mildly. (The CARET study does not slow me down a bit.)

To give yet another interesting perspective (*Harvard Health Letter*, April 1995, p.11):

> Researchers may have been too quick to assume that beta carotene by itself deserved credit for lower cancer rates, according to nutritional epidemiologist Regina G. Ziegler of the National Cancer Institute. People who ate diets rich in fruits and vegetables or who had high circulating levels of beta carotene showed a reduced risk of cancer. But, she pointed out, "blood levels of beta carotene may simply be a good marker for fruit and vegetable intake."

I am giving extra attention to beta carotene as a prime example of the impressive potential of the carotenoid group. Yet, other representatives of this group which are present in carrots (such as alpha and epsilon carotene), exhibit some or all of the same attributes as beta carotene. For instance, they all show antioxidant, anticancer and immune-enhancing qualities.

Calcium Pectate, Carrot Calcium, and More

Calcium pectate, a type of soluble fiber present in carrots, is showing itself to be yet another fiber with cholesterol-lowering properties. A USDA study found that participants who ate 7 ounces of carrots a day for 3 weeks had an average of 11 percent reduction in cholesterol levels (*Wellness Encyclopedia of Food and Nutrition*, p.75). That sounds like a good result for just 3 weeks of eating a small dose of tasty carrots, don't you think?

Carrots possess a variety of B vitamins as well as several minerals, including a healthy dose of calcium and potassium. In fact, carrots have enough calcium to warrant them being used as a source for a *Carrot Calcium* supplement made by the Dr. Bronner Company, and available at health food stores. Carrots also have a notable amount of folacin, the B vitamin noted for its help in prevention of birth defects, in blood building, and for anti-atherosclerosis activities.

Plainly, carrots deserve their place on my 10 *Essential Foods* list.

Carrot Juice for Life

Since carrots are sweet with natural sugars, they have earned a fine reputation as an energy-enhancing snack food; one that is also easy to carry around, and available almost anywhere in the world. Personally, if my travels take me to places where I have the luxury of getting fresh organic carrot juice when I want it, I consider myself close to paradise!

For healing and rejuvenating purposes, carrots are a major ingredient in the life-giving, fresh vegetable juices used with profound results at some of the most successful so-called "alternative" cancer-healing and general health clinics around the world. (Speaking of clinics, I must put in a short digression: Some of the state-of-the-art "alternative" clinics in the United States, Sweden and in Tiajuana, Mexico are providing a real breath of fresh air—i.e., new found hope for many sick people. The healthcare offered in these clinics often has a stunningly positive effect without damaging the immune system beyond repair, as many of our more "traditional" radiation and chemotherapy methods do! See the Clinics listed in Appendix A.)

Carrot juice, preferably organic (but don't refrain if it isn't), is a viable Addition or Alternative to eating whole carrots for whatever reason—personal enjoyment or as part of a healing regime.

In addition to the common type of carrot/vegetable juicers (in which the juice is spun out of the fiber), a Vita-Mix machine will take any fresh whole fruit or vegetable and liquefy it, fiber and all. This renders a thicker juice that is still a completely whole food, with all its functional components. (With a Vita-Mix machine you can make frozen ice cream-like desserts from whole frozen fruits, grind Brown Rice and other whole grains fresh on the spot for cereals and breads, and quickly make whole-food fresh juices which contain their total nutrition. Besides tasting good and appealing to the "quick, simple and easy" mentality many of us embrace regarding food, the Vita-Mix can play an important role in preparing whole foods for someone convalescing from an illness. See Vita-Mix in Supplies Appendix B, and in my Gadgets list in chapter 2.)

Carrot juice is a concentrated food that is rejuvenating as well as cleansing to the body. The only precaution I offer about drinking carrot juice is that neophyte carrot juice drinkers sometimes overdo it. Four to eight ounces a day is a reasonable amount to start with, and many juice connoisseurs dilute their juice, half and half, with pure water. If you ever feel that drinking carrot juice has given you a slight headache, it is probably because you are drinking more than your body is able to handle at the moment. Lower the amount you drink at any one time and consider diluting it. While veteran juice-drinkers don't hesitate to drink a quart or more of fresh carrot juice a day, I suggest you work up to it. *Intuitive Eating*, by Humbart Santillo, N.D., contains pertinent information about the use of fresh juices for health and healing.

TASOLE: Friends and family are often pleasantly surprised to find that children can be inspired to eat fresh vegetables, and even practically fight for them, under the proper circumstances. One such circumstance, starring carrots, occurred with a group excursion to visit my food-artist friend, Jeremy. (My editor says this story is simply too unbelievable ... but it's her word against mine!)

A curtain was drawn back from the entryway to Jeremy's dining area. Our 15-member group walked in, chattering and carrying on like we always do until every child and adult in our party was silent, awed at what we saw. A moment later the room filled with squeals and giggles of pleasure, as anticipation swept through the crowd. We were looking at a fairyland scene made entirely of fresh fruits and vegetables—featuring knights riding horseback through fields of grass; and clusters of farm animals. Small buildings sat here and there next to a stream. The centerpiece, yet to be uncovered, was veiled under a silvery-blue cloth. The whole scene was perhaps three feet wide and four feet long.

My friend Kate was nearly breathless: "Jeremy even used potatoes and squash to make different shades of skin tone. Look at that green pepper top for a knight's shield and the alfalfa sprouts growing straight up for grass!"

Jeremy gave us about ten minutes to look things over more carefully before he stepped up and took hold of the cloth covering the centerpiece. "The centerpiece is always a special surprise," I told Kate. "Hold up the children so they can see it all."

The cloth swooshed away to reveal a phantasmagorical, two foot long orange dragon, complete with individual scales, detailed claws, wings, teeth, and tongues of friendly-looking flames shooting from its mouth. (There must have been an inner framework, probably of some very light gauge wiring. But we couldn't see those inside parts and I never got around to asking about it.) Nearly every detail of this remarkable creature was made of carrots!

"I never knew carrots came in so many shades of orange and red!" exclaimed one of the adults. (The children simply gasped "Wow!") Indeed some of the shades were as light as pale peach, and I wondered, skeptically yet silently, if Jeremy had bleached them.

"Just carving each scale must have taken hours," someone else remarked, as we all circled around the dragon, examining it and wondering how it was all held together.

The exquisite wings were made of carrots sliced lengthwise so thinly we could see through them like a shimmering orange cellophane. The dragon's fingernails and toenails were of reddish carrots affixed to dark orange carrot toes and fingers. The "scales" of the head were of lighter shades of carrot, gradually moving into darker, more vibrant tones towards the tail.

The entire scene was so spectacular that we temporarily forgot what Jeremy considered our main reason for being there—we were expected to eat it all!

At first we were a little timid. But then, "I want a piece of the wing," shouted one child. "Give me a shield (green pepper) from a knight, and a spear (celery)," called another. I decided to start with a plate of dragon scales (carrots) and pond water (vegetable dip). Others went for a boat (banana) and oars (mango). And there were several near-blows when, on a few occasions, two children wanted the same vegetable-character or prop.

"I never knew my children could or would eat so many fresh fruits and vegetables," Kate commented as we sat on my porch later that evening. "That carrot dragon has captured their imaginations so much that I think they want to try and make one of their own for tomorrow's dinner."

As the years passed I lost touch with Jeremy; he got invited to travel around demonstrating his food art. But, I still can't look at a carrot anymore without thinking of that incredible carrot dragon.

"TOO MANY CARROTS?"

Carrot and carrot-juice lovers have occasionally asked me if one can eat too many carrots? I say yes. Though carotenoids, including beta carotene, are non-toxic and highly useful antioxidants for our health, eating too much of them can cause the skin to turn shades of yellow or orange. In medical terminology this harmless condition is called *carotenemia*; and it only affects the skin. (If the whites of the eyes were to turn yellow, or the urine become discolored, for instance, this could indicate an unrelated health problem for which you should see a health-care professional.)

Some people can begin accumulating beta carotene under the skin causing yellow to orange pigmentation to occur. This occurs with ingestion rates above approximately 30 mg. beta carotene (sometimes referred to as 50,000 IU's) per day (beta carotene being the strongest coloring carotenoid and most likely to cause this phenomena). Thirty mg. of beta carotene a day, solely from carrots, could amount to eating about two or three medium-size carrots every day for probably more than a couple of weeks—beta carotene absorption varies from person to person and food source to food source. So, "too much" in this case doesn't mean a near-death experience, but one could change colors temporarily until it wears off with a few days of not eating carrots.

I find the "orange skin" scenario more commonly happens amongst those who drink two or more glasses of carrot juice every day for weeks at a time, although I have known many such drinkers who have not a hint of yellow even after years of such consumption. Anyway, beta carotene from dietary food sources is not dangerous, in fact is highly desirable. But, if you notice an unwanted orange tinge to your skin, it might be time to slow down or stop your carrot consumption for awhile.

SHOPPING FOR CARROTS and OTHER FOOD SKILLS

Fresh organic carrots are always best, but remember, you can detoxify the regular store-bought carrots when you must (see instructions for detoxifying in chapter 2). Fresh, crisp, non-organic carrots might be better than old, wilted yet organic ones.

Have you ever noticed how the bags containing carrots at many grocery stores have thin orange lines printed on them or a dark band printed around the bottom? These are marketing tricks to give the illusion of brighter, fresher-looking carrots, or to hide the stem ends of the carrots so it is harder for a shopper to check those ends for clues to optimal liveliness. Whether you are buying carrots in a bag or not, gently try to bend them to check for firmness (they should not be wimpy and bendable). Check for the darkest orange color, don't settle for yellowish ones; and check the stem ends as best you can for discolorations or softness indicating spoilage.

To get the most beta carotene value out of your carrots they should be lightly cooked (steaming or cooking with a minimal amount of water so that the carrots remain rather crispy). (Note: a pudding-like mush is not the same as "lightly cooked.") However, if you need mashed or puréed carrots for a recipe, it works well to lightly cook them and *then* mash or purée them in a food processor, getting the best of both worlds. Light cooking dramatically enhances the absorption of the beta carotene (by several times) in your body. The cooking slightly breaks down of some of the carrot fiber and increases the digestibility of certain components of the carrot which are locked into those fibers. Cooking can, however, lessen some of the other more heat-sensitive nutrients and enzymes of carrots, but, I must report that I am amongst the first to eat any roasted carrots I am offered, knowing full well that roasting is well beyond "lightly cooked." Roasted carrots still have some nutrition left in them; and when I'm in the roasted carrot mood I don't care about all the rest.

Don't peel your carrots before eating or cooking, whenever the choice is up to you. The peels contain such a concentration of nutrients it would probably be smarter to eat the peels and throw the rest of the carrot out if you absolutely had to make such a heart-wrenching choice (which I hope you never do).

HEALTHY ADDITIONS, ALTERNATIVES and TRAVELERS TIPS

Any deep-orange to red root vegetables, such as red or yellow beets, would be a fine Alternative to carrots. Great Additions would be all the other vegetables in the orange/red range such as red chard, purple cabbage, rhubarb or red radish.

For long-term storage, traveling and camping, properly dehydrated carrots are a profitable Alternative to fresh carrots. Frozen carrots are also OK and can still provide some good nutrition even though they would be my third choice behind fresh or properly dehydrated carrots. You might even find frozen carrots at a health food store that still have their peels intact.

As a travel food, carrots can usually be found anywhere in the world, even open air markets in out of the way places like Nepal, and the wilds of Mexico or South America. If you can't detox them while traveling in such places, peeling them would be a good choice because of the high prevalence of air-born contaminants, such as parasites, in certain areas. Carrots are usually available at restaurants in various guises. Even if they are not on the menu, you can usually get steamed or roasted carrots for the asking. Salad bars with any intelligence will always have raw carrots available.

For those who want the health benefits of living foods but find that their lifestyle often creates obstacles to acquiring or preparing foods, "live food" supplements are the answer. (Also invaluable for children who need more vegetables in their diets.) Two of the best I have found are *Phyt-Aloe* (chewable or capsule) sold through mail-order by Rejenitec Company, and whole leaf *Wheat Grass*, or *Barley Grass* produced by the Pines Company. (See more information in the Healthy Additions section of chapter 4, Broccoli; and also in Supplies Appendix B.)

SURVIVAL CHOICES for COMPROMISING CIRCUMSTANCES

Canned carrots might be better than none at all. And just in case you "survivalists" are wondering—Carrot Cake does not count for much in the carrot-nutrition department, although for taste you surely have a point.

KIDS LOVE THIS

Put on your orange tee-shirt and serve up a fresh carrot salad—made from grated carrots mixed with juicy raisins which have been soaked in water for awhile. Add a little of the extra soak water from the raisins after mixing up this salad. Sweet and delicious.

Another not-to-be-missed recipe:

GINGERED CARROT MARMALADE

1 cup grated carrots
2 Tbs. water
3/4 unpeeled organic lemon, sliced (remove seeds)
1 1/2 to 2 tsp. minced ginger
1/2 cup honey
1 Tbs. pure pectin (no sugar or chemicals)
2 Tbs. water

Put the carrots, lemon, ginger and water into a blender. Blend to a coarse mixture. Put the mixture in a bowl. Add the honey and pectin. Mix well. Refrigerate 3 hours, or overnight.

NOTE: If you don't like ginger, just eliminate it for a delicious Carrot-Honey marmalade.

Recipe from: Nostrand, Carol. *Junk Food to Real Food* (New Caanan, CT: Keats Publishing, 1994, p. 197). Used with permission.

DULSE-SPROUT SALAD

1/2 cup dulse quickly rinsed and drained
2 cups any Sprouts (1 3/4 cups alfalfa and 1/4 cup lentil are a good mix)
1/4 cup scallions chopped
1/4 cup red sweet peppers, chopped
1/4 cup celery, chopped
1/4 cup avocado, chopped

Toss all these ingredients with your favorite salad dressing or add 1 tsp. lemon juice and 1 tsp. soy sauce [or *Bragg's Liquid Aminos* (see Supplies Appendix B)].

Recipe from: *Maine Coast Sea Vegetable Recipes.* Franklin, ME: Maine Coast Sea Vegetable Company, 1996. (1-207-565-2907, or lots of great information through their E-mail: mcsv@acadia.net)

FUNCTIONAL COMPONENTS
In 7 Grams Dried Dulse. (Because dulse is so extremely light in weight compared to other foods, I have decided to list functional components in 7 grams, or one serving, instead of the usual listing for 100 grams. This will make the data more meaningful. So, even though the numbers may appear quite small, remember that the components are in their most available form; therefore quite potent and significantly useful in each serving.)

Serving Size: 1/3 cup dried dulse (approximately 1/4 oz. or 7 grams)

Calories	19.0
Protein	2.0 g
Fat	.12 g
Carbohydrates	3.12 g
Fiber	2.3 g
Cholesterol	0
Calcium	15.0 mg
Phosphorus	29.0 mg
Magnesium	19.0 mg
Potassium	547.0 mg
Sodium	122.0 mg
Iron	2.32 mg
Iodine	.36 mg
Copper	.03 mg
Manganese	.08 mg
Zinc	.20 mg
Selenium	yes
Fluoride	.37 mg
Chromium	.01 mg
Vitamin A	46.40 mg
Vitamin C	.41 mg
Vitamin B1 (Thiamin)	.01 mg
Vitamin B2 (Riboflavin)	.13 mg
Vitamin B3 (Niacin)	.13 mg
Vitamin B6	.63 mg
Vitamin B12	.50 mg
Vitamin E	.12 IU

Prominent Phytochemicals and Antioxidants in Dulse:
Vitamin C, vitamin E, beta-carotene, algin.
Source: Independent laboratory analysis for Maine Coast Sea Vegetable Company in Franklin, Maine (see Appendix B).

7

DULSE

AND OTHER SEA VEGETABLES

WHAT IS SO GOOD ABOUT DULSE?

Dulse and all sea vegetables have no equals in the plant kingdom when it comes to major mineral and trace mineral content. They are so nutrient-rich that a little bit goes a long way. Sea vegetables also contain some phytochemicals which are unique to ocean-grown plants. (Throughout this chapter I will use the terms "ocean" and "sea" interchangeably.) In addition to this, sea vegetables are one of few documented non-animal dietary sources of vitamin B12, an essential nutrient.

A Sampling of Nutritional Factors in Sea Vegetables

The carefully analyzed information that follows is taken from a variety of experts, including the Maine Coast Sea Vegetable Company (MCSV), an organically certified sea vegetable harvester and purveyor located on the northeastern shores of the U.S., since 1971 (see Supplies Appendix B). Their dulse, along with three other types of edible sea vegetables growing naturally on the coast (alaria, kelp, and laver/nori), are available all over the U.S. at health food stores and even some grocery stores.

Sea vegetables contain:

- **Vitamin B12**—one of few documented non-animal sources, especially important for vegetarians. Although dulse has good vitamin B12, laver has 2 1/2 times more.
- High amounts of **iron**—One 1/4 ounce serving of dulse or kelp gives up to 30% of the RDA, 4 times the amount of iron in Spinach.
- Impressive amounts of non-dairy **calcium**—A serving of alaria delivers the same calcium as 1/2 cup cottage cheese, 1/3 cup yogurt, or 3 servings of cream cheese. The same serving contains more calcium than 1/2 cup boiled kale or boc choy.
- Substantial amounts of **potassium**—A serving of kelp contains almost twice as much potassium as a banana, and about as much as one potato.
- A significant source of **chromium**—which helps regulate blood sugar, especially important to diabetics and hypoglycemics. Kelp and alaria are especially high in chromium. Adequate dietary chromium may help prevent adult-onset diabetes.
- Kelp's **glutamic acid**—A natural "MSG," this amino acid tenderizes peas and legumes and makes them more digestible. (I always cook a hunk of kelp or alaria in any pot of beans for a surprising improvement in flavor, nutrition and digestibility.)
- Phytochemicals, like **alginate (algin),** found only in sea vegetables—are compounds which may account for the traditional use of sea vegetables in Oriental medicine. They are used for their antitumor, antibacterial, antiviral, antitoxin, and hypocholesteric properties. Algin is a natural gel in sea vegetables, particularly kelp, which is also used commercially in everyday items such a ice cream, pudding, medicines and salad dressings.
- Live **enzymes**—Raw food eaters and others seeking "living foods" find sea vegetables enzyme-active. And the ones from Maine Coast Sea Vegetable Company are all dried in the sun or in special drying sheds at low temperature.
- Full range of **major and trace minerals**—in a form easy for the human body to assimilate.
- An excellent source of **iodine**—especially in kelp. Sea vegetables eliminate the dietary need for seafoods (which are high in iodine), or iodized table salt. Thyroid medication should be adjusted accordingly.

- **Vitamin K**—important for blood clotting. Dulse is one of the highest sources of vitamin K of any food group, containing 120 mcg per 1/4 ounce serving.
- Small amounts of high quality **protein**—with an excellent protein:calorie ratio. Dulse and laver offer about 2 grams per 1/4 ounce serving.
- **Vitamin E**—Alaria and laver are highest in vitamin E of the four sea vegetables considered here. These two contain about twice as much vitamin E as dulse.
- **Beta carotene**—Alaria and laver have as much or more beta carotene per gram as fresh Broccoli, Spinach and many other top rated greens.

LALITHA RANTS: *Mentioning calcium, as I did in the list above, has got me thinking about what I consider to be some common misinformation. For those who follow the conventional medical advice of eating over-the-counter, chewable, calcium-based antacids as a cheap calcium source, be warned! Many of these products, have calcium, yes. But this type of calcium neutralizes your stomach acid (which is the job it is made for). Yet, without stomach acid working, no calcium can be broken down and absorbed; nor can many other nutrients. My observation is that this type of calcium simply "gums up" your digestion, and your health, in the long run. As calcium supplements go, these antacids are worse than no calcium at all!*

Only take those antacids when you absolutely need an anti-acid. Why won't doctors who still believe in that stuff as a calcium supplement get a life! Or rather, update their education about nutrition! Don't they know they do more harm than good with their prehistoric "eat-anti-acids-for-a-calcium-supplement" advice?

And while I'm on the subject ... avoid calcium supplements made from chalk (calcium carbonate), egg shells, oyster shells, and rocks (dolomite)! You might as well be trying to make some kind of permanent sculpture inside yourself when you eat those things!

If you need extra calcium, get it from the *10 Esssential Foods* along with the Additions and Alternatives whenever possible. If you need further supplementation for special health reasons, see my suggestions under Calcium, in Supplies Appendix B.

JOURNEY TO THE BOTTOM OF THE SEA

When you get through this chapter you may feel as if you have been through a science fiction story—that is how vast the difference is between vegetables of the ocean and vegetables of the land. Sea plants have been around for thousands of years, which makes them some of the oldest species of plants on earth. Technically, they are types of algae. Sea vegetables derive nutrition directly from water into their leaves etc., rather than from soils and then through root systems as land plants do.

Most sea vegetables attach to the ocean bottom with *holdfasts*, rootlike organs that cling to rocks. But these holdfasts are not food gatherers. They are simply mechanical devices that hold plants in place so they don't get ripped away during tides and storms. Some kinds of sea vegetables are *free floaters*. A sea plant can "hold fast" to the bottom, forty feet below, while having a major top part of the plant floating on the surface of the water gathering sunlight for photosynthesis.

With plants grown in the mineral-rich ocean there is never a crop failure, or poor growth due to lack of nutrients or drought. Minerals eroded from the land wash down to the sea, constantly enriching the food supply there. Cold ocean currents tend to be richest for supporting the most wildlife and the teeming growth of sea vegetation, while tropical water are somewhat less productive.

Sea vegetables are prolific growers. Kelp can grow up to two feet a day in the summer and many types of sea vegetables renew their tissues several times a year. This amount of production rivals and often surpasses some of the most productive land crops. (For more on this subject see: *Food Power From the Sea*, by Lee Fryer and Dick Simmons. New York, NY: Mason/Charter, 1977.)

To anyone living in a coastal area, "seaweed" may be no stranger, but *eating* seaweed may be an entirely different story. To the majority of Americans, at least, eating sea vegetables regularly as a health-enhancing food source, probably seems akin to eating chocolate-covered ants. Nevertheless, the information in this chapter bears so strongly on the information in all the other chapters and relates so significantly to building or maintaining vibrant health, that I consider it to be the most basic and critical knowledge for health building. Therefore, I will never stop urging you to put aside any previously learned resistance to this possibly "new" food. Teach yourself and your children that sea vegetables are definitely "in" as a regular and enjoyable part of your diet.

TASOLE: "Tamara won't like that," Joan said to me as I was about to offer a snack to her five-year-old daughter Tamara. Tamara and Joan were visiting me just as I was about to have an afternoon energy-boosting bite of dulse, a lovely burgundy-red-colored sea vegetable that is naturally salty-tasting and crunchy. It tastes mildly of the fresh ocean.

"She's a very picky eater and doesn't like unusual foods," repeated Joan while eyeing my dulse suspiciously.

"Lots of kids love this stuff," I said, somewhat defensive of one of my favorite snacks.

"I want some," repeated Tamara as she reached for the bag of dulse.

Tamara popped a bit of dulse into her mouth and began sucking and chewing on it—tentatively at first and then quite enthusiastically. Then, with a smile, she reached for another bit of dulse while Joan looked on with a mystified expression.

I held out the bag to Joan who reluctantly put a small piece into her mouth. She too was soon smiling with enjoyment.

I thought to myself, "I bet it's not really Tamara who's the original picky eater in the family."

As often happens, dulse slowly infiltrated that family's diet as one member after another insisted on trying "that red stuff Lalitha gives to Tamara."

THE B12 DILEMMA

Within nutritional circles the question of whether or not a person can get enough vitamin B12 from non-animal sources, or absorb enough in any case from animal or plant sources (many people are deficient whether they eat animal products or not), often causes a lot of fuss; and not without good reason. Vitamin B12 is vital in maintaining the health of the nervous system which generates the electrical signals necessary to run every operation in the body. Vitamin B12 is crucial for memory function, for the processes of carbohydrate, fat and protein metabolism and is essential for the formation of blood cells.

Without it we can expect to be forgetful, nervous, tired, anemic and (at worst) even brain damaged.

In his book *Intuitive Eating*, author Humbart "Smokey" Santillo, N.D. states that Vitamin B12 "... is not made by plants and animals, but by a bacteria the plants and animals contain. Humans have B12 throughout the body—between the teeth, in the gums, tonsils, and saliva. [*Some*] B12 is produced in the small intestine [*by friendly bacteria*]." (p.192)

Part of the B12 dilemma is this: while generous amounts of vitamin B12 are available from animal products, many experts say that ingesting these animal products will mean taking in a significantly health-negative amount of concentrated protein and fat, not to mention the contaminants in these foods. Santillo, among others, concludes that non-vegetarians need extra amounts of nutrients, such as B12, to counterbalance the effects of eating animal products. This, in turn, has contributed to a faulty calculation of how much vitamin B12 a vegetarian would really need.

Exactly how much of this crucial vitamin B12 is truly needed in the diet for vegetarians and for non-vegetarians? Medical and nutritional researchers agree it is a tiny amount. Just how tiny an amount is graphically described by Michael Colgan, Ph.D., in his book *The New Nutrition: Medicine for the Millennium* (Ronkonkoma, NY: Advanced Research Press, 1994, p.32). Colgan writes:

> You require only a few micrograms (millionths of a gram) of B12 a day: the RDA [*our government's "recommended daily allowance"*] is only 2 micrograms. Your blood contains only about 5 nanograms (billionths of a gram) per liter, less than a speck of dust.

Colgan goes on to point out, however, that without those crucial nanograms of B12 one quickly develops symptoms from anemia to insanity!

According to Santillo, who also quotes the agreement of several of his colleagues, vegetarians need only .5 micrograms of added dietary B12 a day (yes, that is point five) to maintain optimal health. Humbart Santillo, N.D., says that the criteria for amounts of B12 needed in vegetarians and non-vegetarians is different partly due to the differences in their protein intake, as I mentioned previously. Also, vegetarians tend to absorb B12 better than non-vegetarians, and vegetarians seem to have a higher production of vitamin B12 going on in their intestines, perhaps because of the larger colonies of friendly bacteria happily lodged there.

Another highly respected researcher, Alexander Schauss, Ph.D., senior director of research at the Southwest College of Naturopathic Medicine, has specifically and thoroughly investigated optimal intake levels for vitamin B12 and recommends 2 mcg. per day. (Schauss, A..G., Ph.D. "Establishing a suggested optimal nutrient allowance. Cyanocobalamin, Vitamin B12." In: Pizzorno, Joesph, E.,*Textbook of Natural Medicine.* Seattle, WA: John Bastyr College Publications, 1992.)

Continuing on in our research we find that, in their best-seller nutrition book, *Prescription for Nutritional Healing* (Garden City Park, NY: Avery Publishing, 1990), Phyllis A. Balch, C.N.C. and James F. Balch, M.D. place the Optimum Daily Allowance (ODA) for B12 at 300 mcg! (To my knowledge, no toxic levels for B12 have been found.) The ODA amounts are educated "guesstimates" indicating how much of a nutrient would promote optimal health, rather than the RDA amount which will simply prevent the "drop dead" symptoms of bad health. However, neither the ODAs nor the RDAs take into account whether a person is a vegetarian or not.

Obviously, there is no unamimous agreement about vitamin B12 intake other than that it is crucial to good health. There can be no guarantees of optimal health, whether or not you are vegetarian and whether or not you are getting a lower or higher amount of B12. Common sense tells us that there are endless complexities to maintaining the chemical balance among all the functional components that result in optimal health.

Whether we decide we need *more or less* B12, there is no question that we *do* need it. And dulse and other sea vegetables are at the top of the list of vegetarian sources for vitamin B12. (Even though what I call the "old school" nutritionists still stubbornly claim there is no B12 in any plant food!) In addition to sea vegetables, other vegetarian sources of B12 are nutritional yeast and fermented vegetarian foods such as sauerkraut, miso and tempeh (these last two are delicious fermented soybean foods available at your health food store). These types of fermented foods depend on the use of bacteria for fermentation and these bacteria are producing B12 as they do their jobs. This is also true for "live culture" yogurt. I always try to buy *unpasteurized* fermented products whenever possible because pasteurization kills the friendly bacteria in these "live" fermentation cultures, thereby lessening the B12 content along with other nutrients and active enzymes.

For myself, in addition to these foods mentioned above I supplement with tablets of a highly nutritious fresh-water algae (fresh-water vegetable) called *Klamath Blue-Green Algae* (see Supplies Appendix B). This algae, from fresh-water Klamath Lake, is a whole food that contains vitamin B12 as well as many other amino acids, antioxidants, chlorophyll and nutrients that help keep me going in spite of who-knows-what. It has several properties in common with the vegetables we harvest from the oceans and is perfect for someone like me who prefers to get nutrients from whole foods whenever possible.

Dulse and all of these vitamin B12 vegetables are vital components of the *10 Essential Foods* system.

MINERALS—TRACE and OTHERWISE

Because of the type, variety and amounts of major minerals and trace minerals contained in dulse and other sea vegetables, these should be considered extremely important foods. At least 70 different major and trace minerals are found in dulse and sea vegetables—minerals which help maintain vibrant health in ways known to science (and in many ways as yet unknown). Just as with vitamin B12, trace minerals are present in the human body in minute or "trace" amounts, and yet without them our quality of life slips away from us as body and mind degenerate. The importance of minerals to health and vitality cannot be overstated or overemphasized, but I will spend several pages of text giving it my best try. If you really grasp what I will describe to you about minerals, you may have to catch your breath with the wonder and shocking possibilities of it all.

Ionic Minerals Mean Life

An ion is an electrically charged particle. A mineral ion, electrically charged either positively or negatively, is the smallest particle a mineral can exist in. Mineral ions are the form that minerals must take to be absorbed by our cells for use in the body's life processes.

The minerals in our bodies, which are used predominantly in liquid ionic form (also called electrolytes), are vital catalysts and carriers of the energy within us—chemical energy, mechanical, electro-magnetic, or electrical energy. From an electrical point of view, the human body runs on electricity.

Literally. A legal definition of death is when all electrical activity in the brain has ceased. If we say, "I wish I had more energy," or "I'm running out of energy," we are actually referring to our inability to conduct electrical impulses/messages (energy) adequately throughout our bodies.

To oversimplify how the human electrical energy system works, major mineral and trace mineral ions (with positive or negative electrical charges) create electricity in the body through a positive/negative, attraction/repulsion process as they move within body fluids across cell membranes. Consider neurons, for example, which are the conducting cells of the nervous system. Neurons communicate with one another, without physically touching, via the flow of charged ion particles from cell to cell within body fluids. In going from cell to cell as quickly as thought, these (mineral) ion-facilitated impulses continually repeat, or propagate, electrical "messages" that are sent all over the body to govern and facilitate *all* of its functions, including muscle movement, heart beat, endocrine activity and creative thought.

Lest we underestimate this process, remember that even picking your teeth, never mind competing in an Olympic marathon or writing the great American novel, depends on the body's electrical ability, which depends on minerals. And of course, in order for us to enjoy the flavor of the 10 *Essential Foods* we must have the electrical conductivity that depends on major and trace minerals *in their ionic form* in our bodies.

Where do we get ionic minerals in our diet?

Top sources for ionic minerals are fruits and vegetables (sea vegetables being at the top of the list). Fruits and veggies also contain highly available food-bound forms of minerals which quickly become ionic through digestive processes. While there are minerals in almost all of the foods we eat, the plant kingdom is a source for those with high bio-availability, in their easy-to-digest form.

In addition to foods, water can be a significant source of many trace elements, whether ionic or not. Many people have access to pure, mineral-rich water from springs or wells, for instance, and in many places there are now "water stores" from which one can often purchase water with its mineral content undiminished (reverse osmosis and distilled waters have the minerals removed). However, even though the mineral content of the right type of water can certainly contribute significantly to our health, a possible problem is acquiring pure water free from the chemicals and other contaminants which proliferate in most public water supplies, while maintaining the mineral integrity.

The smart consumer will insist on pure water with its trace elements still present, and will go to the extra trouble to get it—even if this means buying a household water filter which removes contaminants but not the minerals, buying pure water by the gallon, or signing up with a reputable "water store" for regular delivery of pure water to your home and office.

Since the subject of water—its purity, sources, minerals content, water filtering systems, etc.—is a huge one, I am not going to delve into it in any further depth in *10 Essential Foods* (perhaps another book is called for). However, under Water Filters in Supplies Appendix B, I do point the way to the best water filters.

For myself, knowing that trace mineral content of most foods and water is quite variable, I depend upon an ionic trace mineral supplement, in addition to sea vegetables and a good diet, to insure that I am getting the full range of trace minerals needed for optimal performance. (See Trace Minerals in Supplies Appendix B.)

When traveling, even if I am buying the best bottled water a country has to offer, I know that scientific analysis shows these waters are almost always deficient in important trace minerals. I add several drops of my mineral supplement to any water I buy because I don't want to experience the sad difference (weakened health) without them!

What To Do With All These Minerals

Minerals produce enzymes by the thousands, and enzymes facilitate the function, absorption and utilization of vitamins and other functional components. Without minerals, vitamins are useless, period. Vitamins and other functional components in turn are essential in the production of hormones, digestive fluids, brain chemistry, fertility, emotions, mood—you name it. Without minerals, and minerals in proper amounts and in balance with one another (trace minerals do not exist by themselves but in relationship to one another), that legal definition of death which I mentioned earlier becomes either slowly or quickly apparent in each of our cases. We may call it an eating disorder, arthritis, bad moods, depression, cancer, ulcers, diabetes or aging but "a spade is a spade." At bottom, mineral deficiencies are mineral deficiencies! Much evidence, scientific and otherwise, supports this idea that minerals are the foundation of health.

Alexander Schauss, Ph.D., author of over fifty health-related publications, including *Minerals, Trace Elements and Human Health* (Tacoma, WA: Life Sciences Press, 1996), research psychologist and mental health therapist, as well as Senior Director of Research, Southwest College of Naturopathic Medicine and Health Sciences, Tempe, AZ, tells of his extensive work with patients suffering from *bulimia nervosa* (binge-purge behavior), *anorexia nervosa* (self-induced starvation), or morbid obesity. In almost every case a zinc deficiency is found to be directly involved. For instance, Schauss found that the lower the zinc status, the more morbidly obese the individual. In patients with osteoporosis, Schauss explains that no matter how much calcium and magnesium is given, these patients simply do not respond until the trace mineral boron is added. Boron facilitates the maintenance of calcium in the bone, reduces urine excretion of calcium, magnesium and phosphorus, and significantly increases estrogen and testosterone in blood serum. Both estrogen and testosterone hormones are important in calcium absorption.

Elderly patients with low mental functioning improve when the trace mineral selenium is given, Schauss reports. Selenium protects the heart and boosts the immune system. (Sea vegetables are a top source for selenium.) The mineral lithium contributes to stable mood when it is sufficiently present and (indirectly) to manic-depression when it is lacking. People exhibiting violent behavior have higher than normal amounts of manganese in their systems, and often high amounts of toxic metals as well. Dr. Schauss has significant clinical and research experience proving the causative/curative role that mineral balance plays in social/criminal behavior. Fascinating information on this topic of behavior and minerals can be heard on the audio cassette of a lecture he gave in July 1994 entitled: *The Role of Essential Trace Elements in Human Health and Behavior.* (This lecture was given at the annual tradeshow of the National Nutritional Foods Association and is available through Tree Farm Cassettes, 1-800-468-0464.)

A Future in Minerals?

Since plants absorb minerals from the soil, the condition of our soil is of vital concern for the health of future generations.

As far back as 1936, the U.S. Senate was warning of the extreme depletion of minerals from our soils.

Excerpt from U.S. Senate Document #264
(Published by the 2nd session of the 74th congress 1936)

Do you know that most of us today are suffering from certain dangerous diet deficiencies which cannot be remedied until the depleted soils from which our foods come are brought into proper mineral balance?

Laboratory tests prove that the fruits, the vegetables, the grains, the eggs, and even the milk and the meats of today are not what they were a few generations ago (which doubtless explains why our forefathers thrived on a selection of foods that would starve us!)

No man of today can eat enough fruits and vegetables to supply his stomach with the mineral salts he requires for perfect health, because his stomach isn't big enough to hold them.

It is bad news to learn from our leading authorities that 99% of the American people are deficient in these minerals, and that a marked deficiency in any one of the more important minerals actually results in disease. Any upset of the balance, any considerable lack of one or another element, however microscopic the body requirement might be, and we sicken, suffer, and shorten our lives.

Lacking vitamins, the system can make some use of minerals, but lacking minerals, vitamins are useless.

More recently, in June of 1992, an Earth Summit meeting in Rio de Janairo addressed environmental factors all over the world. Almost all world governments were represented. The Earth Summit Report clearly showed the devastating and increasing decline of mineral values in farm and range soils all over the world. North America (U.S., Canada, and Mexico) was by far the most seriously affected,. with South America, Asia and Europe not far behind.

LALITHA RANTS: *Folks, what this means in plain language is that most of the produce we find in American markets is, as far as mineral content is concerned, "looking good and going nowhere." What do those experts mean that our minerals have been leaving our soils for over 60 to 100 years! Where can a mineral go anyway? What about matter being neither created nor destroyed? Huh? Those minerals have got to be somewhere.*

So what? you ask. So maybe we have been kicking and sucking them out of our soils for over a century without properly replacing them? We've got to grow lots of food somehow, and fast, don't we? Well, don't we?

North America is the worst ... and we still pride ourselves on being the best farmers. Think about this for a minute. Water goes up, evaporation, la la la, water comes down, plants draw minerals up from the depths of soil, then minerals are easily washed away, lee lee lo, erosion, mountains crumble, water runs to the sea, la dee da, THE SEA! That's it! That's where all those minerals are going!

Where's my bag of dulse? I never want to be without my sea vegetables again!

The mineral content of the *10 Essential Foods* is impressive. In fact, the *10 Essential Foods* are some of the highest-rated fruits and vegetables, where minerals are concerned. You will still assure yourself enormously better health in eating these foods than if you don't. Yet, except for dulse and other sea vegetables, the nutrient potential of even the other 9 *Essentials* is steadily lessening compared with what it has been in the past, or what it can be again and is now, with organic farming methods. The soil-mineral depletion created by "modern," non-organic farming methods, coupled with the replacement of only a few selected minerals in a diet of highly-processed foods, has left most Americans deficient in major and trace minerals, and therefore victim to myriad modern degenerative diseases.

Other factors affect the mineral depletion of our soils as well. Soil erosion, for instance, increases with more aggressive farming methods and/or harsh climatic conditions. Many fertilizers and pesticides bind trace minerals in the soil so that fewer minerals are absorbed by fruits and vegetables. Do you see what I mean about the seriousness of the situation we are in?

Our oceans and seas are constantly collecting and recycling extensive concentrations of the full range of the minerals that are being washed back into them through the processes of nature. Dulse and other sea vegetables, grown in this mineral-dense environment of the ocean, pick up these functional components and prepare them within their own tissues into a food-form fantastically suited for our diet. Additionally, sea minerals, coupled with sunlight and decaying sea life, and catalyzed by forces not available on land, contribute to the production of phytochemicals and antioxidants in the sea vegetables—a few of the reasons why, for centuries, sea plants have been used with great success in Oriental medicine for health maintenance, rejuvenation and healing. Unfortunately, the majority of data supporting this success is not yet translated into English.

Do We Need to Take a Mineral Supplement, or Not?

As I have described, most Americans have significant mineral deficiencies, especially of trace minerals. While we can more easily replenish our major mineral supply through dietary sources (barring specific illnesses such as osteoporosis which generally require mineral supplementation), it is often a smart idea to take a trace mineral supplement *in addition to* having sea vegetables in the diet. (Remember, supplements cannot replace the complex nutrition of all the functional components available in whole foods.)

But, what supplement should you take?

After having researched the subject extensively (and believe me I am good at it), it is obvious that many mineral supplements are minimally absorbed in the human body because of the form of minerals used. Other factors, such as age, adequate amount of stomach acid to break down minerals, overall intestinal health and dietary fiber intake, also influence your ability to absorb minerals.

Regarding mineral supplements, there are lots of terms thrown around—including organic/inorganic, metallic, colloidal, electrolyte, chelated, coated, bound/unbound and ionic—to convince consumers of the usefulness (absorbability) of various *forms* of mineral products. Some companies seem to ignore form altogether and simply sell (in any form that suits their market) what I consider to be highly un-assimilable *sources* of plain calcium—such as oyster shells, rocks (dolomite), egg shells, "plaster of Paris" (calcium sulfate) and chalk (calcium carbonate)—with the implication that neither the form nor the source makes any difference. (Some doctors even recommend simply using the cheapest source/form of calcium you can find, no matter what it is.) Such marketing angles can be very confusing, especially when everyone says the "other guy's" products are not good enough.

Remembering that ionic is the form in which our bodies use minerals, an important question about a supplement becomes: "Can this mineral supplement be easily digested into ionic form?" For the poor sources I mentioned above my opinion is definitely NO! The good news is that we consumers can buy many minerals already in their ionic form and nevermind all the marketing maze and questions about whether or not a supplement will break down properly. (See Minerals in Supplies Appendix B.)

HEALING PROPERTIES OF DULSE AND OTHER SEA VEGETABLES

At least one American researcher has looked into the health and healing properties of seaweed. Jane Teas, of the Interdisciplinary Programs in Health, Harvard School of Public Health, Boston, MA, published a study entitled: *The Consumption of Seaweed as a Protective Factor in the Etiology of Breast Cancer.* (See Recommended Bibliography.) The abstract reads:

> A review of the biological properties of seaweed is presented and the role of seaweed as a breast cancer anti-carcinogen is suggested. Proposed mechanisms of action are: reduction of plasma cholesterol, binding of biliary steroids, inhibition of carcinogenic fecal flora, binding of pollutants, stimulation of the immune system, and the protective effect of beta-sitosterols. In an experiment using sarcoma-180 in mice, seaweed extract appeared to have an antitumor effect. Thus it is suggested that breast cancer may be prevented and that this dietary habit among the Japanese could be an important factor in understanding the lower breast cancer rates reported in Japan.

In *Prescription for Cooking* (Greenfield, IN: PAB Books Publishing, 1987), authors Phyllis A. Balch, C.N.C. and James F.

Balch, M.D., devote a whole section to sea vegetables, including a review of world research on the healing properties and preparation. The Balchs report that the sea vegetables with the darkest leaves, such as kelp, kombu (an Atlantic form of kelp), wakame and hiziki, all contain alginic acid (algin) which can convert toxic heavy metals in the body into harmless salts that are easily discharged. Accumulation of (toxic) heavy metals is implicated in Alzheimer's disease and many other "unexplainable" health problems.

Sea vegetables have quite a reputation for preserving health in the face of radiation poisoning, whether the radiation is the result of medical treatments, "natural" atmospheric pollution, or nuclear fall-out. After the A-bomb, Japanese medical personnel saved many radiation-poisoned victims by administering a diet of miso soup, Brown Rice, and sea vegetables! At McGill University in Canada, researchers found that the dark sea vegetables can remove radioactive strontium-90 from the body. I know many health professionals who suggest a daily intake of kelp tablets, powder, or liquid, or other dark sea vegetables in some form, for protection from chemotherapy, radiation and x-rays. Along these lines, in August of 1996 I came across a Wire Service article (vol. 27) about the Hadassah-Hebrew University Medical Center near Tel Aviv where, through administering beta carotene from Red Sea algae (seaweed from the Red Sea), dramatic and positive results were found in treating children poisoned from the 1986 Chernobyl nuclear accident. I thought of dulse, which is a deep dark-red sea algae high in beta carotene. Dulse is specifically acclaimed as being one of the most nutritious sea vegetables, containing all 43 trace minerals.

As I explained in the Introduction, the color of a plant points to its array of phytochemicals and antioxidants (important in the actions mentioned in the abstracts above). The kaleidoscopic colors of ocean plants, such as the deep burgundy red of dulse, indicate a food source of invaluable benefit for humans.

THE SALT QUESTION

Many people ask, "Isn't the sea salt associated with sea vegetables dangerous to one's health?" The answer is, almost never. Except for renal patients, and those suffering from severe hypertension and CHF, most people can enjoy sea vegetables in varying amounts, sea salt and all. The sodium in sea vegetables is balanced with calcium, magnesium and potassium, making it a far "different animal" than the sodium chloride of table salt. In fact, many folks have switched to using sea vegetable seasonings (available from MCSV and other companies) instead of table salt on their food, thereby lowering their blood pressure and gaining other health advantages, while still getting great taste in their food! After independent laboratory analysis, Maine Coast Sea Vegetable company found that:

- A serving of dulse has one half to one third the sodium found in one cup of most breakfast cereals, and less sodium than one slice of most commercial breads.
- One cup of cooked beet greens has as much sodium as two or three servings of dulse.
- The sodium content of an average sea vegetable serving is often less than that of a carrot, a serving of chard, or a bagel.
- Compare the sodium in 1/4 ounce of sea vegetables to the sodium in 1/2 teaspoon table salt. Kelp has 1/3 as much sodium, Alaria 1/4, Dulse 1/8, and Laver 1/9!

In an official note to health professionals, Maine Coast Sea Vegetable experts write:

> Even patients on modified clinical diets can healthfully incorporate moderate to liberal amounts of sea vegetables; just remind them to limit their intake of [*salty condiments such as*] shoyu, tamari, miso and processed foods. For patients on a no-added-salt diet (about 2500 mg), sea vegetables can give just the right saltiness, and are far better in nutrition and taste than commercial "lite" salts. Used in moderation, they can be enjoyed in a typical serving of 5 to 10 grams (about 1/4 ounce).

In any case, you can always lessen the already small amount of sodium on sea vegetables by simply rinsing the vegetable before eating.

TASOLE: "Here's a question for you ... "
This is how David often began his sessions of consulting with me about the best dietary choices for his year-round camp/retreat center for adults as well as children.

The camp focused on creative expression, including poetry writing, weaving, stained glass, painting and drawing, to mention a few activities. One of the additional specialties of this camp was that the food was renowned for being healthy and rejuvenating as well as tasting so great that both the children and the adults loved it. In particular, David enjoyed serving up healthy snacks to his camp participants.

In our meetings, he and I played an unspoken game—he would describe the ideal results he would like, all packaged up in one food if possible, and then I would be challenged to come up with a creative solution.

"I want to add more trace minerals to the camp diet, possibly in the form of a snack, or perhaps a new food, but I don't want it to be sweet," David began. "It is OK if it is a little bit salty, but not oily and cheesy like most junk food, and it wouldn't hurt if it was colorful." He took a breath and thought for a moment. "In order to be able to fit into camp activities, I want it to be lightweight and require no special storage temperature or preparation. I like turning my campers onto something new when they come here. New food ideas they will want to take home."

"Are you talking about all the same snack? Or, ten different choices?" I laughed as I interrupted him. I was well aware that he took his camp-food menu very seriously, but this description really got me smiling. I was certain he thought that finally he had come up with a description which did not fit anything good-tasting yet healthy I had ever heard of.

"I want it all in one snack, of course!" he smiled back. "In June, which starts our big summer season, we'll have lots of campers here and that's when we have our camp food-testing week. We offer different new foods at every meal and then ask the campers to vote on them. The high-rated ones get added to the menu. As you can imagine the snack department always attracts a lot of interest, to put it mildly."

"How about dulse?" I offered. "It has every quality you mentioned plus some."

"Can you think of anything else?" David asked. "I know you mentioned that a couple of years ago. It's that red-looking seaweed isn't it? Er ..."

I raised my eyebrows at him as best I could (I can't do it very well but it was definitely called for). "Are you saying you've never tried it yet, even after two years?"

He looked a little embarrassed. "You're right. I didn't take that suggestion of yours very seriously. I've never had sea vegetables of any type on the diet here because I guess I thought that most people would find them too unusual. Now that you are mentioning it again, though, I remember that sea vegetables are part of Japanese cuisine, and lots of people love Japanese food. But I thought that seaweed took special skill in preparation. Can this dulse really fit into my description?"

"Let's put it into the food testing try-outs during June in several different ways," I offered. "I'll work with the food preparation staff. You'll see."

During food try-out week, all new offerings were put out with a number as an identifier. There were "food helpers" always available to describe in general the qualities of an item without directly divulging exact ingredients. (That way no one could simply say, as David might have, that she wouldn't want to taste an item because she "probably wouldn't like a sea vegetable," before even trying one.)

"Sure, let's do it," David agreed. "This should be especially interesting."

Amongst the huge variety of new items offered during the food week I had arranged for four different soups, two pots of beans, two vegetable sautés, and three fresh salads offered at different times which all included dulse in a significant way. The condiment table always held a shaker of dulse powder (to sprinkle on food), and a bowl of plain, dried dulse to munch on was always available on the snack table.

These food try-outs were in actuality a week long food feast with so many dishes offered that one had to pace oneself in order to taste a majority of items. All participants were enthusiastic and highly critical judges and voters. Many had come this particular week for this specific event—never mind any other creative activities!

Each evening, when the day's foods were voted on by number, many participants, including David, became fairly rowdy, vigorously lobbying for their favorites. One night early in the week David told me excitedly, "I'm making a big push for today's soup; and yesterday my favorite salad won! This is great fun!"

It was not unusual to see an adult or child hopping up and down shouting, "Yes for number 23! Come on 23!" like they were at a horse race or something. Or conversely, "No on 12! Nobody vote for that one!"

Once the voting was over the menu winners were announced, and their ingredients listed. Needless to say, many people were stunned to learn that they had voted for an item that contained dulse, a sea vegetable. And by weeks end there was a wonderful cornucopia of new additions to the camp diet for the year.

"I should have listened to you two years ago," David admitted with a sheepish grin. "My favorite soup, the vegetable mixture I voted for, and that red stuff in the shaker which I added to my rice, all turned out to be dulse dishes! Lots of other people voted the bean salad marinade to the top of the list, and it had lots of dulse in it too."

"What about the snack table? What were the winners there?" I asked, knowing full well that the children had a major say-so in that area.

"That was the biggest surprise of all," David reported. "Even regulars who have been coming to this food week for years didn't guess the outcome on that one. Banana chips got a big thumbs up along with the Fig bars ... those weren't so unexpected. But the dulse was a regular dark horse. It was a little sneaky of you, Lalitha, to put it out every day, instead of just once or twice. But, by the end of the week I could see why you did it."

"Well ... ah ... some items are so new for some people that they take getting used to," I began warily. "Did you notice how people kept coming back to try the plain dried dulse again each day, even though at first they weren't sure why they liked it?"

David was visibly enthusiastic. "That dulse got more votes each day. Even the kids were stuffing a handful into their pockets when they went off to other activities. In fact, from what I heard, it was the kids who lobbied most to make dulse one of the top three snacks of the week. I never would have guessed it. Have you got any other weird ideas you'd like to suggest ... for next year?"

SHOPPING FOR SEA VEGETABLES and OTHER FOOD SKILLS

Even with sea vegetables it pays to buy from an organically certified source. As you know, many ocean areas around the world have become heavily polluted and issues of how, when, where, and how much is harvested, as well as how the plants are transported, dried, stored and packaged are important to consider. Good sources for quality sea vegetables include Eden Foods and Maine Coast Sea Vegetables (MCSV). I know that MCSV is organically certified, and that they test their dried plants for the absence of heavy metals, herbicides, pesticides, and microbiological contaminants. Sea vegetables harvested from ocean sources in other parts of the world may or may not be harvested from clean waters or handled according to environmentally-positive practices which will ensure a continued and uncontaminated supply. MCSV sells only those sea vegetables—including dulse, alaria, laver, and kelp—that naturally grow on their northeastern U.S. coast. Eden Foods sells sea vegetable choices from other parts of the world. I use both companies regularly. (See Supplies Appendix B.)

Whether you cook sea vegetables or not, you can hardly hurt their mineral content. They can be toasted, boiled, stir fried, sautéed, pickled, marinated, bought in a ground-up form and used as a sprinkled seasoning; or in the case of dulse, eaten raw right from the bag. Sea vegetables can be added into soups, salads, sandwiches or whole grains and are delicious in fish and meat dishes.

I take a small handful of dulse, very lightly rinse it under water (to soften it), squeeze out the excess water and lay it on my plate as a condiment to be added to any food I am eating. What I end up with on my plate are beautiful, soft, tender, red dulse leaves which are easily picked apart with my fork and added to various items. Sometimes I just put the dry dulse next to my dressed salad where it soaks in the extra salad dressing. Then I eat it as an "instantly marinated" delicacy by itself or with other foods. Also, I always keep a shaker of dulse powder on hand to sprinkle as a seasoning onto foods during or after cooking. Dulse powder gives a salty-type flavor, while actually providing a very minimal salt intake.

Whenever I make split pea soup, or cook a pot of beans, I put in several large handfuls of dark green alaria (a kelp-type sea vegetable). After my slow-cook-for-several-hours method of bean preparation (this means I like to put the items in the pot with lots of water and come back later to eat, with no fuss in between), the alaria has "melted" completed away into the food leaving a wonderful flavor, texture and digestibility with nary a leaf in sight. This is a great way to get sea vegetables into the diets of sea-vegetable-newcomers who always become admirers after tasting such a delicious dish.

Since dulse and other sea vegetables may be new to some of the readers of *10 Essential Foods*, you may want to rely on some cookbook ideas to help you take full advantage of the possibilities. (See: Cookbooks, in the Recommended Bibliography for several listings.) In addition, any library should have Japanese cookbooks which will definitely call for sea vegetables. Macrobiotic cookbooks offer another source for prolific sea vegetable recipes.

The Maine Coast Sea Vegetable company also offers a collection of recipes for dulse and all their other sea vegetables (call them at (207) 565-2907 to order a copy). Even though dulse is tasty right out of the bag, you will want to develop a variety of "sea vegetable habits" and these recipes are the way to go. At health food stores you will also find other great tasting MCSV products such as *Sea Seasonings, Sea Chips, Sea Pickles, and Maine Coast Crunch*, a lightly sweet, crunchy and chewy snack bar made with kelp.

HEALTHY ADDITIONS, ALTERNATIVES and TRAVELERS TIPS

While dulse is the star of this chapter, any sea vegetables are suitable Alternatives. Others that I especially like are arame, nori, and hiziki; all fairly mild yet with outstanding flavor. Although they are not sea vegetables, other mineral-rich Additions to the diet are Figs (giving even sea vegetables good competition in the case of calcium, potassium, magnesium), kale, Broccoli, chard and all cruciferous vegetables.

When traveling, it is easy to inconspicuously carry along a bag of dulse for snacking. Dulse travels very well, has a years-long shelf life, and is a perfect light-weight nutritional Addition for any trip or camp out.

Another "traveling choice" is to buy dulse or kelp tablets at your health food store. With a sea vegetable tablet, you can get a serving of sea vegetable by taking a few of them at any meal, whether that be in a restaurant or under mosquito netting in the jungles of Mexico!

SURVIVAL CHOICE for COMPROMISING CIRCUMSTANCES

If you can't get sea vegetables, you may be able to find Oriental-style frozen dinners which contain them. Also, although shellfish can have a high contamination factor, they do "grow" in the ocean as do sea vegetables and they do contain minerals. So, in compromising circumstances, a serving of shellfish such as shrimp, oysters or lobster might suffice.

KIDS LOVE THIS

Children usually go for dulse plain, fresh out of the bag, if given an unbiased chance to do so by the presiding adult. Also, roasting/toasting dulse in a dry pan on the stove top, or in the oven, makes a crispy nibble that children and adults will definitely desire more of.

Additional Recipes:

QUICK DULSE SOUP
Something fast that's not "fast food."

3 1/2 cups boiling water
1 onion chopped
1 cup dulse chopped
1 cup parsley chopped

First add the chopped onions to the boiling water. A minute later add the dulse and parsley (or finely grated Carrot, daikon, cabbage, etc.), cover and turn off heat. Add soy sauce, miso [or *Bragg's Liquid Aminos* to taste (see Supplies Appendix B)]. Serves 3.

SPINACH WITH DULSE

Steam together 8 ounces frozen Spinach or 2 full cups fresh Spinach with 1 small, sliced zucchini or summer squash. Rinse 1/4 to 1/2 cup dulse and cut to desired bite-size pieces. Dice 1 or 2 cloves of garlic and sauté in a very small amount of olive oil for about 1 minute, adding pinches of basil, cumin, and cilantro. Add the dulse and sauté 1 or 2 minutes more. Remove from heat and add the juice of 1/4 to 1/2 lemon. Pour over steamed Spinach and zucchini and serve. Serves 2.

DULSE/GARLIC POPCORN

Toss freshly popped corn with melted butter [or *Barlean's Flax Oil*]. Sprinkle on *Dulse/Garlic Sea Seasoning* liberally, and toss again. *Nori/Ginger Sea Seasoning* also tastes great here. (*Sea Seasonings* are from the Maine Coast Sea Vegetable Company.)

Recipes from: *Maine Coast Sea Vegetable Recipes*. Franklin, ME: Maine Coast Sea Vegetable Company, 1996. 1-207-565-2907. Lots of great information is available through their E-mail address: mcsv@acadia.net

HEARTY FIG OATBRAN MUFFINS

1 1/2 cups bran flakes cereal
1/2 cup apple juice
1 egg
1/2 cup non-fat milk
6 ounces apple juice concentrate
3 Tbs. olive oil
1 large banana, mashed
3/4 cup figs, finely chopped
2 Tbs. honey
1 1/2 cups oat flour or whole wheat flour
1/2 cup oatmeal (rolled oats)
1 tsp. cinnamon
1 1/2 tsp. baking soda
2 tsp. baking powder

Combine your favorite bran flakes in a large bowl with the apple juice. Moisten the flakes evenly. Add the egg, milk, apple juice concentrate, oil, banana, figs and honey. Mix well. In a small bowl, combine flour, oatmeal, cinnamon, baking soda and baking powder. Add to bran mixture and mix well. Line a muffin tin with paper liners. Spoon batter into paper lined muffin cups. Bake at 350 for 20 minutes or until done. Yield: 12 muffins

(Also see the recipe for Mediterranean Chicken and Figs in Chapter 13)

Recipe from: California Fig Advisory Board, 3425 N. First St., Suite 109, Fresno, CA 93726. 1-209-445-5626. Used with permission.

FUNCTIONAL COMPONENTS

In 100 Grams Dried Figs
Serving Size: approximately 3.5 oz, or 1/3 cup, or 100 grams, or 6 to 9, dried, uncooked figs.

Calories	282.0
Protein	3.05 g
Fat	.5 g
Carbohydrates	65.35 g
Fiber (including soluble)	12.0 g
Cholesterol	0
Calcium	144.0 mg
Phosphorus	68.0 mg
Magnesium	59.0 mg
Potassium	712.0 mg
Sodium	11.0 mg
Iron	3.05 mg
Copper	.313 mg
Manganese	.338 mg
Zinc	.51 mg
Selenium	yes
Chromium	30.0 mcg
Vitamin A	133.0 mg
Vitamin C	.8 mg
Vitamin B1 (Thiamin)	.071 mg
Vitamin B2 (Riboflavin)	.088 mg
Vitamin B3 (Niacin)	.694 mg
Vitamin B6	.224 mg
Folacin	7.5 mcg
Vitamin B12	0
Pantothenic Acid (Vit. B5)	.435 mg
Vitamin E	0
Biotin	yes

Prominent Phytochemicals and Antioxidants in Figs:
zinc, vitamin A, ficin, benzaldehyde, psoralenes.

Sources:
1) Santillo, Humbart, N.D. *Intuitive Eating* (Prescott, AZ: Hohm Press, 1993).
2) California Fig Advisory Board, 3425 N. First St., Suite 109, Fresno, CA 93726. 1-209-445-5626

8

FIGS

WHAT IS SO GOOD ABOUT FIGS?

Figs! The solar energy fruit! In addition to the impressive information about the functional components of figs that fills this chapter, I must also point out a major contributing factor to the power of figs (admittedly somewhat subjective on my part) which is often highly undervalued by more conventional sources of data. This component is sunlight. It is well known by scientists and lay people alike that all life in nature, including human life, depends on the sun for existence. We have all experienced this, at least intuitively, during those times on a sunny day when we step outside, take a deep breath, sigh contentedly, and say, "That sun sure feels good."

Dr. Johanna Budwig, a German physicist, medical doctor, author and seven-time Nobel Prize nominee has lectured and researched extensively why this sunlight phenomenon is objectively true—i.e., why humans are literally antennas for sunlight. During one of Dr. Budwig's lectures ("The Fat Syndrome and the Photons of Solar Energy," 8th *Vie et Action* Congress, Tours, France, April 6, 1972) when she was discussing the benefits of Flaxseed oil, she also emphasized that, "The electrons from our foods act as a resonance system for solar energy. Electrons derived from foods are real nutrients. They attract the photons of sunlight with their electromagnetic field." Dr. Budwig explained that humans and foods can therefore become storehouses for the life-giving photons of sunlight.

Being a highly intuitive sort myself, I have determined that figs are a wonderful source of these photon-attracting electrons, partly because figs need to interact with the sun concentratedly at every stage of their development. Figs are sun grown, sun ripened, sun dried and sun filled. Even though this may be true of some other dried fruits, raisins for example, when this sunlight attribute is added to the unique functional components of figs, this fruit earns its place on the *10 Essential Foods* list.

FIGS ARE ... FIGS HAVE ...

For you food enthusiasts who like fig facts that can be measured, here are a few to titillate you.

- Figs have the highest dietary fiber content of any common fruit, nut, or vegetable. (Dietary fiber 40% higher than raisin bran!)
- Figs are up to 1000% higher in calcium than other common fruits; 133 mg in 3.5 ounces. (In fact, on an equal weight basis, figs have a higher calcium content than whole milk.)
- Figs are over 50% higher in potassium content than bananas (generally thought of as the best source).
- Figs have plant protein content nearly twice as high as other dried fruits and over ten times that of most fresh fruits.
- Figs have a high content of easily digestible natural sugars such as glucose and fructose.
- Figs have a higher overall score in mineral content, including trace minerals, than other common fruits.
- Figs have a natural humectant to extend shelf life or freshness of baked items.
- Figs have a lower calorie count per gram of dietary fiber than other popular fruits, and even lower than nearly all of the highly promoted bran cereals.
- Figs have only 20 to 40 calories per fig, depending on the size of the fig.
- Figs are higher in pectic fiber than other fruits. This soft soluble fiber helps the body remove toxic waste and reduces the cholesterol level.
- Figs are virtually cholesterol, fat and sodium free.

Allow me to translate some of these functional, famous, fabulous, fig facts into practical terms. Dietary fiber, soluble and insoluble, has been shown to help prevent colon cancer. Dietary fiber keeps bowels moving, thereby preventing or relieving constipation; lowers cholesterol thereby contributing to heart health; and helps shrink hemorrhoids and colon polyps (polyps are often a pre-cancerous condition).

Potassium is important in nerve functioning, fluid balance, muscle contraction and heart rhythm. A diet containing adequate potassium can lower blood pressure and drastically cut the odds of suffering a stroke (for a diet rich in the *10 Essential Foods* this amount of potassium is simply supplied by six figs a day, or 1/2 cup cooked Spinach, or 2 Carrots, or 2 ounces of Almonds).

The different types of sugars in figs are an efficient fuel for an active person. These types of sugars burn slowly, giving a sustained-release effect unlike the fast-burn, quick-crash, poor health syndrome associated with processed sugar junk foods. All things considered, there is no reason ever again to follow the junk food monster down his old rutted road called "Get Fat—Feel Tired—Ruin Your Health."

WHERE FIGS ARE FROM

In the United States, all of the figs commercially grown for dried figs come from California, predominantly from the San Joaquin valley. The climate there has much in common with the hot dry climate of the Mediterranean from where our fig varieties were first imported.

In learning how figs were harvested in California I was pleased to find out that, for the most part, figs are allowed to fully ripen on the trees. When they fall off the trees, it is harvest time! You may remember, from the Introduction, that in judging the quality of fresh food it is an asset when food can fully ripen before harvest, thereby encouraging the fullest availability of functional components, many of which do not even occur unless the fruit or vegetable is allowed to grow to maturity.

Apparently, the fig industry tried several times to invent harvesting equipment similar to that for other fruits such as plums. Automated harvesting means that the trees are shaken by a machine, causing both ripe and unripe fruit to fall off into a canvas collector. The fruit is then encouraged to ripen the rest of the way by various means. Such methods put the growers in charge of the timing, and fig growers desired such a plan.

Fortunately for us, however, no suitable method was ever found for automated harvesting of those delicate-skinned figs, which would land with a splat on the harvesting canvas and be ruined. Early clipping by hand was also tried, to rush the harvest, but this was also a failure. Finally, the growers had to accept that the best plan was to sit back and wait for the figs to fully mature and partially dry right on the trees. When figs are partially dry their skins are a little tougher, so when they naturally fall off it is a happy ending to their growth cycle; and yet another reason why figs are unique among fruits.

The two major fig varieties grown are Calimyrna figs, a beautiful light-skinned fruit and Black Mission figs, delectable deep purple-black beauties. However, home-grown varieties of figs are many and they grow under such a wide variety of circumstances that fig trees can be found in virtually every state, if not every town in the country from Alaska to Florida! I was pleasantly surprised to find that there was a fig grower not far from my own small Arizona town. I discovered this when his tasty fresh figs began to show up in limited supply at my local organic produce store. What a find! I must have been such an obvious fresh fig fanatic that even the store manager noticed. (This might have been because, upon discovering these organic beauties, I audibly squealed—I had thought tactfully and hopefully invisibly—with delight. After this the store manager began calling me whenever he got a delivery. If you squeal properly you might be able to set up a deal like this too!)

Figs win a prize for what is *not* done to them. Figs are rarely sprayed with any pesticides! This is a markedly different circumstance than is the case for most other dried fruits; raisins, for example, are highly treated with pesticides and preservatives from the beginning to the end of their growth and production process, unless they are organically grown. It turns out that the hot and dry climate of the San Joaquin valley, where U.S. figs are grown, provides a natural insect control for figs. Apparently the only time a pesticide spray is called for is after a summer rain between July and October. (Spraying is deemed necessary when damp fruits start to ferment on the ground, creating a very attractive aroma for insects which will then spoil the remaining ripening fruit, if not taken care of.) However, a rain during these months is unusual—approximately once every ten years! Ron Klamm (pronounced Klumm), Manager of the California Fig Advisory Board for over thirty years, told me that as far as he knows "no California fig grower even owns a spray rig!"

In addition, figs do not need to be preserved with the toxic waxes and fungicides common to many other fruits. Figs grown for dried fig use do need a mold inhibitor because they have a high moisture content and would develop disastrous mold problems after processing. For this, potassium sorbate is sprayed onto them following a hot water washing. Potassium sorbate is a preservative well known for its safety on foods and for which no toxicity levels have been found.

The only other process that might happen to a fig being readied for market is the possibility of being sulfured. Sulfur (sulfite) preservatives, usually in the form of sulfur dioxide, are used with many light-colored dried fruits, such as apricots, bananas, apples or pineapple to preserve their color. The food may be looking pretty because of this treatment but a smart consumer doesn't want to eat sulfites. These preservatives can produce allergic reactions, sometimes extreme—asthmatics are often especially sensitive. But, whether we notice an immediate sensitivity or not, sulfites accumulate in our bodies contributing to health chaos later.

Since manufacturers are required to list preservatives on their product labels, all we have to do is look for word "unsulfured." Calimyrna figs, being light-skinned fruits, are often sulfured, yet not always, as modern refrigerated storage has lessened the need for it. Black Mission figs, being dark-skinned fruits, are never sulfured; no need for it. Aside from organic figs of every sort, Black Mission figs are always my favorite choice for taste, texture, safety and nutrition.

THE MIRACULOUS PHYTOCHEMICALS

Figs contain commercially significant amounts of some highly useful enzymes and phytochemicals. Ficin, a protolytic enzyme contained in figs, is active in digesting proteins from either plant or animal sources. Figs are therefore quite useful as a before or after meal digestive helper. In fact, several digestive enzyme products depend on figs as a primary ingredient. Ficin also contributes to an enzyme combination in figs which, along with a type of fig phytochemical called psoralenes, helps bring about beneficial results in skin injuries, in removal of dead skin tissue (for example in cosmetic uses such as facial scrubs), in cases of vertiligo (a skin disease involving lack of pigmentation in patches of skin), and for possible uses in vaccine research. In fact, an Associated Press article dated April 12, 1989 reported that psoralenes from figs were used in ancient Babylon (4000 BC) in treating skin pigmentation diseases.

For me, an even more exciting phytochemical found in figs is benzaldehyde. I first heard of this phytochemical from sources at the California Fig Advisory Board. Subsequently, this long name caught my eye in other places. The prestigious *Townsend Newsletter for Doctors* (October 1991) summed up everything I had so far come across. Basically the scoop is that benzaldehyde was being used by Japanese and Norwegian researchers as far back as 1985 with positive results in the prevention and treatment of cancerous tumors.

An anecdotal tidbit I heard from Mr. Klamm at the Fig Advisory Board concerned a French medical doctor and researcher, Dr. Bordeaux, who discovered that radioactive particles in figs prevented growth of cancer cells and curtailed cancer growth. This was not the first time I had uncovered brief reference to this finding of "radioactive particles" in figs having exciting health and healing activity. Perhaps someone who knows more details about this property of figs will write to me in care of my publisher.

In serving an eleven-year apprenticeship in the usage of medicinal plants (see my book *10 Essential Herbs*), I learned of several internal and external applications for figs that correspond to these findings of the conventional research literature. Of course, in those days I didn't know why a fig poultice worked for skin ailments, or for drawing infection to a head, or why eating figs enhanced bowel action, digestive efficiency and provided energy. All I knew was that figs worked, were great food, and had a flavor that was almost universally liked.

TASOLE: My friend Pam told me one day of her continual struggle with leg cramps and a vague ache in her hip which kept her awake at night and dragged down her energy during the day.

"Lalitha," Pam said, "I have been to that local chiropractor who is always able to magically fix structural 'glitches,' and he says nothing is pinched or out-of-alignment. He suggested I might have a nutritional deficiency, even though I eat a good diet."

As Pam spoke I recalled that she was still nursing a young child and that she was also quite physically active. "So, did he suggest a supplement or anything?" I asked.

"He recommended calcium and magnesium and I have been trying them, in different forms and amounts, taking them at night, taking them in the morning ... But it's frustrating. I'm getting some relief but not quite enough yet. What do you think is the missing link?"

Of course I had what I thought was a brilliant idea. "Have you tried eating a few figs every day?" I asked. "It doesn't matter if they are fresh or dried," I added.

"Figs? I love figs!" Pam responded enthusiastically. Then she laughed, "No, I haven't eaten any lately, but what has that got to do with my problem?"

"I don't want to give you a whole lecture about figs," I replied, without sounding too impatient. "You can look up all the details about them at the library if you're interested. But, suffice it to say that figs are quite high in specific nutrients such as calcium (more and better than milk!), magnesium, phosphorus, potassium, copper and iron. All these substances soothe nerves, strengthen body tissues and prevent muscle cramping. My healing teacher regularly gave Black Mission figs to the three of her twelve children who were active in school athletics. She knew that figs would prevent cramps and therefore lessen the possibility of injury. She told me that figs had a range of trace minerals that helped absorption of other minerals and nutrients."

Pam was skeptical. "It could have been a coincidence. Her children might have been fine even if they didn't eat the figs," she said.

"As a new apprentice, I thought so too, at first," I countered. "Then I began to study nutrition more. Now I have learned about the enzymes, nutrients and plant chemicals available in figs that can account for all these positive effects. Even at that time, however, the team coach caught onto the fig idea when it quickly became clear that my teacher's children healed faster, had less cramping and did not injure as easily as their team-mates. When the coach started encouraging the whole team to eat figs, it made a noticeable difference for everybody. I think your body too might be happier with getting the nutrients it needs from figs," I told Pam. "Figs are simply more 'alive' than vitamin pills. Try about five figs a day."

A month later Pam called and reported that she had "incredible" results with the figs after only two days. No more mysterious aches and pains! And the figs really helped her energy level. As long as Pam kept figs in her daily diet she felt great. If a day or two went by without the figs, even if she took a calcium/magnesium supplement, the problem slowly started returning. When she stopped breastfeeding her child, Pam's body only needed two or three figs a day instead of the recommended five. But, she didn't slow down. Why should she! She loved those figs!

SHOPPING FOR FIGS and OTHER FOOD SKILLS

When choosing dried figs, make a serious effort to get unsulfured ones for reasons described above. If you can't be sure, then go for the dark skinned figs, such as Mission figs, as these don't need sulfur to keep their color. Whether fresh or dried, it is always preferable to buy organic when possible. Non-organic fresh figs (or any fresh fruit) can be "detoxed" (see chapter 2), but this is a little tricky with fresh figs because they are so extremely delicate and perishable that during the detox process they are easily damaged. Cleaning figs just before eating them is probably the best for fresh figs, to lessen spoilage from bruising that may occur from even careful handling. Since figs are contaminated so little in their processing, there is less to worry about here than with some other fruits.

Many consumers do not buy organic fruits even though non-organic fruits are usually highly contaminated with health-damaging chemicals. This is well-documented in one of my favorite and most up-to-date resources, *The Safe Shopper's Bible* (see Recommended Bibliography). According to that resource, when buying non-organic fruits at the usual grocery store, those with the least risk of serious contamination are apricots, bananas, coconut, citrus, dried peaches (not fresh), prunes, dates and watermelon. (There's a more complete list of minimal risk buys in *The Safe Shopper's Bible* along with well-documented details of contaminants in many other fresh foods.) Some of the non-organic fruits we buy the most—apples and grapes for example—are commonly contaminated with seven to ten serious carcinogens such as azinphos-methyl, captan, dicofol/kelthane, dimethoate, and propargite. Many shoppers pretend that the usual apples off the shelf are just fine.

LALITHA RANTS: *What are all those shiny, sometimes oily, definitely waxy-feeling substances on grocery store fruits and vegetables anyway? Anything that keeps the outer skin of a fresh food*

perfectly great-looking, almost indefinitely—well, any intelligent observer has got to wonder what goes on when that stuff hits your stomach and then heads for your liver. Yeah, sure, the food has got to be preserved somehow, doesn't it?

Well, doesn't it?

If you are talking about one of those apples which is full of contaminants anyway, the preservatives are simply holding in the "bad news" a lot longer. Have you ever bitten into one of those so-called "preserved" apples that look inviting on the outside? You crunch through the plastic-feeling skin only to find an off-color, unappetizing, mushy middle when you follow through on that first big bite. I once bit into an apple skin that was so stiff with wax that a piece of that skin stuck between my teeth hard enough to make my gums bleed; and let me tell you, there is nothing wrong with my gums! Healthy gums, that's what I have! It took two pieces of dental floss to pry that apple skin out of there. Another time, cucumbers at a local market were so slippery with an oily substance that a shopper would practically have had to use solvent to get it off.

So, what do we do? We peel off the skins, that's what we do.

Forced to peel off most of the nutrients—that's what is happening to us when we buy that stuff. Those sprayed-on preservatives must be highly questionable because even my local store has put up large signs trying to explain all that goo. Do they think we will feel comforted by seeing in writing what amounts to a big announcement that petrochemicals and fungicide-containing "food-grade" wax are sprayed on the foods they want us to buy?

I don't feel "protected" by the FDA, that is for sure! Most kids nowadays probably think that those waxes and oils grow naturally on produce skins!

A routine for lessening the risk from contaminants is to be sure to wash and/or detox fresh fruits and vegetables before eating them. Yes, I know I am repeating myself about the detoxing, but it can certainly make a difference.

The easiest way to chop dried figs is to use scissors to cut them. When scissors become sticky, simply run them under hot water. After opening a bag of figs, store it in the refrigerator to preserve the fig's excellent taste.

HEALTHY ADDITIONS, ALTERNATIVES and TRAVELERS TIPS

For Alternatives containing some similar attributes to figs try, unsulfured papaya, pineapple, or mango, fresh or dried. These three especially can contain different yet potent digestive enzymes as well as other notable functional components. For example, papaya which contains the protein-digesting enzyme, papain, also contains the enzyme carpain, which is valuable to the heart and may help relieve heart pain.

Any organic fruit, whether fresh, or dried and unsulfured, can be considered a worthy Addition to figs in a healthy diet. If an Alternative or Addition you choose is not organic, you can upgrade the situation somewhat by using the detox and cleaning methods described in chapter 2.

Since figs, especially the dark skinned ones, have very little contaminants associated with them, they make the perfect buy for a traveler's food in countries with modern agricultural practices. The only hazard I have ever heard regarding dried fruit as a traveler's purchase, is that drying methods in "third world" countries with high concentrations of animal dung in the air, or other unsanitary situations in the environment, may encourage a concentration of contaminants on dried foods. When I am in such a situation, I may buy the dried fruit and then soak it in the Nutribiotic® disinfecting solution I describe in the Grapefruit chapter and in chapter 2.

When traveling (whether it is just to your office, or around the world), and unable to get organic fruit or to properly wash fresh fruit, peeling your fruit is a valuable lesson to learn. This measure will lessen the amount of non-systemic contaminants you consume even though some nutrition will be sacrificed. Dried fruit is easy to take with you on the road, and fruit in general, dried or not, is available at most quick stops on the highway. Restaurants today commonly have fresh fruit in their salad bars. But if you don't see it, chances are they have some fresh fruit in the kitchen for the asking.

A favorite snack of mine, which I often keep at my desk, is *Papaya John's Energy Bars*. A top ingredient in this "miracle food" is figs, but Papaya John doesn't stop there! This bar is full of other energy-producing fruits and foods such as bee pollen and, of course, papaya. Read all about these in the 10 Essential Snacks Appendix C.

SURVIVAL CHOICES for COMPROMISING CIRCUMSTANCES

Fig bars (fig paste wrapped in a cookie-type covering—you know, *Fig Newtons*) from the cookie section of the grocery store could be a Survival Choice if you can't get fresh or dried plain figs. Also, if you or a family member are in the category of, "I never eat fruit plain but I know I like cookies," you can start off with the fig bars as a temporary measure while developing a taste for the "real thing"—the figs themselves. While fig paste *could* be a healthy food and is used in many confections, it can easily have unhealthy substances added to it along with extra sugar. Therefore, it is an item for the Survival list but not my first choice.

Another Survival Choice for fruits in general would be to get simple, unsweetened, frozen fruits of various types. Try to avoid canned fruits as, in addition to their commonly added sweeteners, they usually contain preservatives and their nutrients are much depleted through the additional processing they endure.

Friendly Warning

When adding figs to the diet it is especially wise to add small amounts, slowly. Start with one fig a day and work up from there. Figs help relieve the colon of waste material in such a thorough fashion, that loose bowel movements might result for some people. A capacity for figs will develop easily as time goes on.

KIDS LOVE THIS

In addition to plain figs, children enjoy Fig Balls. Using a food processor pulverize some figs into a paste (or very finely chop and mash with fork and knife if you are energetic and patient) and add pineapple juice as necessary to get a good paste consistency. Usually a very small amount of juice will do. Clean out the processor. (To facilitate the paste-making process, some cooks prefer to soak the figs an hour or two in water or juice prior to mashing.)

Next, grind up a few raw Almonds in the food processor or finely chop them with a knife and add them to the fig paste. Mix thoroughly. (You decide how many Almonds depending on how crunchy or "almondy" you want the fig balls to be. I like about 1 cup figs to 1/8 cup Almonds and I like my Almonds ground to a gritty powder consistency.)

Now you have a sticky paste that can be rolled into balls of whatever size you choose. These Fig Balls may be served as is, or further rolled in unsweetened carob powder or perhaps in dried unsweetened coconut to give a dry outer coating. (Carob powder is a sweet, light to dark brown powder from the carob bean. It has a unique flavor that some find reminiscent of chocolate but it really is in a delicious class of its own and, to my taste, is not like chocolate at all.)

FLAXSEED OIL AND TOFU SPREAD

8 to 10 ounces tofu (try to find a tofu brand that does not contain calcium sulfate, otherwise known as "plaster of Paris" and used in some tofu as a thickener. "Soft" style tofu is more likely to be free of this ingredient.)

2 Tbs. lemon juice or unpasteurized apple cider vinegar
1/4 tsp. dry mustard
1 medium dill pickle, minced
2 Tbs. raw honey
1/8 tsp. minced garlic, or amounts to taste
2 Tbs. flaxseed oil*

Optional: add 1/2 to 1 tsp. each of one or more other fresh or dried herbs such as chives, dill, onion, basil, parsley, or curry to taste. (Using up to 3 tsp. of additional herbs in all.)

Mix together and set aside the minced dill pickle, garlic and flaxseed oil. Do not blend them. Put the other ingredients in a blender or food processor, or blend/mix by hand. Blend until you have a smooth texture. Add the minced pickle, garlic and flaxseed oil.

FUNCTIONAL COMPONENTS

In One Tablespoon Fresh, Unrefined, Organic, Expeller Pressed "High Lignan" Flaxseed Oil
Serving Size: 1 Tablespoon

Total Fat	14.0 g
Saturated Fat	1.0 g
Cholesterol	0
Sodium	0
Calories	115.0
Alpha-Linolenic Acid	
	5600 - 8500 mg (Omega 3)
Linoleic Acid	
	1280 - 1600 mg (Omega 6)
Beta Carotene	132 IU (provitamin A)
Vitamin E	.29 IU (trace amount)
Carbohydrate	2.6% (less than 1 gram)
Protein	1.5 % (less than 1 gram)
Fiber	1%

Other Fatty Acids in one serving include:

Palmitic Acid	5.6%
Stearic Acid	2.4%
Oleic Acid	16%

Minerals: Small amounts of at least 23 minerals important to health.

Prominent Phytochemicals and Antioxidants in Flaxseed Oil:
Vitamin E, lignans, essential fatty acids, beta carotene

Sources:
1) Barlean's Organic Oils Inc., Ferndale, Washington
2) Erdman, Robert, Ph.D. and Jones, Meirion *Fats That Can Save Your Life* (Encinitas, CA: Progressive Health Publishing, 1995).
3) Jade Beutler, author and independent researcher/consultant on Fats and Oils.

This spread can be used as a topping on baked potatoes, other vegetables or whole grains. Good as a vegetable dip, especially with the optional herbs added. Adding more or less tofu will make a more thick or thin texture.

Recipe from Lalitha's kitchen. *Flax Oil recommended is Barlean's.

9

FLAXSEED OIL

WHAT IS SO GOOD ABOUT FLAXSEED OIL?

Flax is a plant that has been cultivated around the world since ancient times. In recent years, flaxseed is getting much attention as a food source which contributes significantly to maintaining good health and rejuvenating poor health. And, lucky for us, fresh, unrefined flaxseed oil tastes enticingly good. World health authorities (such as Michael T. Murray, N.D., author of many books including *The Healing Power of Foods* and co-author of *Encyclopedia of Natural Medicine*; Dr. Johanna Budwig, author of *Flax Oil as a True Aid Against Arthritis, Heart Infarction, Cancer and Other Diseases,* a German biochemist nominated seven times for the Nobel Prize, and recognized as the world's leading authority on the nutrition of fats and oils; and Dr. Robert Erdmann, author of *Fats That Can Save Your Life* and London's foremost alternative health practitioner) all bluntly state the astounding health benefits from adding properly processed flaxseed oil to one's diet. (See the Recommended Bibliography.) Those benefits include the improvement of high blood pressure, arthritis, multiple sclerosis, immuno-suppression, psoriasis and eczema. Flaxseed oil also contributes significantly to the prevention of strokes, heart attacks and cancer, and is used in cancer treatment as well.

The National Cancer Institute in the United States joined the flaxseed bandwagon a few years ago by choosing flaxseed as one of the first and highly-promising foods to be studied in its 20.5 million dollar program to learn more about natural plant chemicals (phytochemicals) that may prevent cancer.

Dr. Budwig's Everyday Miracles

The importance of healthy fats in the diet (flaxseed oil being a most highly regarded one) is dramatically demonstrated by Dr. Johanna Budwig's work in the treating and often curing (yes, curing!) of many types of cancers. Among her seriously ill patients, including those with cancer, she found that without exception they were deficient in one of the essential fatty acids, while the blood of healthy persons always contained sufficient proteins and all the essential fatty acids. While her research shows that protein and essential fatty acids work hand in hand to protect each other, an indispensable and central part of her therapy involves the use of flaxseed oil mixed with cottage cheese or quark (a yogurt-type food) in the diet of the patient.

"Lalitha's short version" of the very detailed information available about how Dr. Budwig's treatments work is as follows. The therapeutic combination of the flaxseed oil with the cottage cheese or quark causes the electron-rich fats (found in high amounts in the flaxseed oil) to become water-soluble through the action of the sulfur-bearing amino acids (components of protein such as cysteine) which are prolific in the cottage cheese or quark. These, now water-soluble, surface-active, electron-rich fats are able to be much more efficiently absorbed by the cells. The body's capacity to activate vital life functions is thus dramatically enhanced, resulting in extraordinary healing and rejuvenating. In addition, and of primary interest to me, Dr. Budwig (as I mentioned in the Fig chapter) has "discovered" that the source of these highly-charged, extraordinarily abundant electrons in flaxseed oil is the sun!

I realize I might be stretching your imagination quite a bit here, but since I have been involved in "alternative healing" adventures my whole life I have, in my own subjective ways, come to the conclusion again and again that the sun plays a profound role in the well-being of humankind. Of course, as a physicist, Dr. Budwig details her findings in ways that are not subjective at all. She demonstrates with certainty that the functional components in flaxseed make it one of the most highly charged foods of all. This is the primary reason why flaxseed oil is one of the *10 Essential Foods*.

You don't have to be sick to reap great benefit from Dr. Budwig's and others' research. Simply include flaxseed oil in your daily diet in whatever way is attractive. A good resource for a large variety of recipes for daily use is *Flax For Life* by Jade Beutler. (See Recommended Bibliography.)

Regarding Dr. Budwig's therapy, most of her books are written in German. Two that I know of in English are: *Flax Oil as a True Aid Against Arthritis, Heart Infarction, Cancer and Other Diseases*, and *The Oil-Protein Diet*. (Both Dr. Budwig's books and Jade Beutler's books are available from the Barlean's Company, 1-800-445-3529, or see the Recommended Bibliography for the complete listing.) Also, there is an American publication, *How To Fight Cancer and Win* by William Fischer (Canfield, OH: Fischer Publishing Corp., 1994) which has extensive information on Dr. Budwig's work plus the work of other highly effective doctors and researchers from around the world.

THE GOOD FAT

Most of us have been bombarded with information about what's wrong with fats and oils in our diets. In fact, I have acquaintances who now have such a fear of fats and oils in their diets that they try to eliminate them altogether, embracing a no-fat diet as much as possible. After reading this chapter, however, you will know why a no-fat approach leads to just as many diseases as the "pack-it-in-and-pass-the-bacon" approach. For me a no-fat diet is out, and the idea of a "right fat diet" is definitely in! Dr. Robert Erdmann (*Fats That Can Save Your Life*, Encinitas, CA: Progressive Health Publishing, 1995, p. 121) describes it this way:

> Healthy fats and oils play active roles at every stage of the life process. They are lubricants, cushions and insulators, guarding against the stresses, concussions and physical extremes that we encounter daily; they are transducers, converting forms of energy such as sound and light into electrical nerve impulses; they provide structural rigidity to cell membranes; and they act as taxis, ferrying harmful substances safely away from sensitive tissue. For these reasons,

[healthy] fat is every bit as important as amino acids, protein, minerals and vitamins.

There are two polyunsaturated fats, linoleic acid (LA) and alpha-linolenic acid (ALA), without which the human body will experience a nightmare of regular breakdown and misfunction. These two fats are basic building blocks for normal cell structure and body function, and are so important they are referred to as *essential fatty acids* (EFAs). As I explained in the Almond chapter, EFAs unlike many other nutrients cannot be manufactured by the body and must be provided in the diet. A diet rich in foods from plant sources is a good beginning toward maintaining intake and balance of these essential fatty acids, whereas a diet high in animal-source foods will take you in an unwanted direction in this regard. Flaxseed oil is an all-star provider of these EFAs.

These two essential fatty acids are often referred to by the name of their general category, i.e., linoleic acid is an omega-6 fatty acid and therefore oils high in LA are often referred to as *omega-6 oils*; alpha-linolenic acid is an omega-3 fatty acid and therefore oils high in ALA are often referred to as *omega-3 oils*. While both categories are crucial to good health, they must be present in the body *in proper balance* with each other as well as in proper amounts. Most researchers describe a healthy balance of omega-6 to omega-3 oils as anywhere from 1:1, to 3 or 4:1. You probably won't be surprised to learn that the balance of these two EFAs in the body of the average American is about 20:1! This basic nutrient imbalance ("way more" omega-6 than is healthy in balance with omega-3) is caused by a diet high in processed and refined foods, grocery store vegetable oils which are highly refined with toxic chemicals, and domestic animal meats. None of these foods are essential for good health. Omega-6 oils *are* absolutely essential, healing and therapeutic, yes; but remember, they have to be in the proper balance with the omega-3's.

LALITHA RANTS: *Omega-6 to omega-3 balance ... that's just one of our problems! I get even more enraged when I think about those grocery store vegetable oils. Don't pay attention to a single additional advertisement about them. Who cares if the advertizers say these bogus oils might raise or lower cholesterol in their unprocessed state. These oils will half-kill you in lots of other ways after processing! It's one of* *those marketing tricks that looks good on paper, but ... Oil manufacturers don't ever tell you that this supposed "good news" about their oils is usually true only before they ruin it! Just thinking of what is usually done to most ordinary oils before we see them at the store gives my liver a big cramp. Solvent-extracted, distilled, another solvent added, degummed, refined, bleached, deodorized, winterized, preserved, defoamed, hydrolyzed, hydrogenated ... you name it! No manufacturer has to tell what they've done to their oil! Why, we'd all be nauseous to the point of vomiting if they did. If the so-called healthy vegetable oils on the market were not processed the way they are, they would smell and taste so bad no one could stomach them. To top it off, we're supposed to believe them when they say that the chemicals from some of these processes are all removed at various stages of this processing nightmare, so we shouldn't worry a bit. Yeah, sure! These oils are toxic, often rancid, indigestible, sludge-producing monstrosities when used in salad dressings, and a million times worse if cooked.*

The average person doesn't have to worry about getting enough omega-6 oils unless he or she has a specific health problem; but almost everyone should consider bolstering his or her intake of omega-3's. Adding at least one tablespoon of properly processed flaxseed oil to our diets on a daily basis can significantly add to the proper balance, because flaxseed oil has a 1:3 omega-6 to omega-3 ratio. (I eat about three tablespoonfuls of flaxseed oil a day, drizzled onto various foods.) Of course, besides adding flaxseed oil I suggest we all go further and begin eliminating all the unhealthy fats and oils along with other processed foods from our diet, while becoming serious fans of the *10 Essential Foods*. The balancing, rebuilding effects on health for everyone who has followed this advice—yes everyone—has been dramatic. (Not the *ho-hum* type of dramatic, where you have to wait a year to maybe feel a small squeak of a difference. I mean a *wocko-socko* can't-miss-it difference!) By eliminating the bulk of unhealthy fats and oils from their diets and focusing on the *10 Essential Foods*, friends have excitedly reported to me that chronic symptoms of ill health, such as joint stiffness, allergies, frequent bouts of flu and other infection, skin problems, or simply general tiredness, just don't happen anymore.

Producing Prostaglandins

One of my flax oil heroes, and a source for much of my data, is Mr. Jade Beutler, licensed health professional, health researcher, and author of *Understanding Fats and Oils, Your Guide To Healing With Essential Fatty Acids*, and *Flax for Life* (both books from, Encinitas, CA: Progressive Health Publ., 1996), along with numerous articles on flax and nutrition. Fatty-acid research is one of Mr. Beutler's pet pursuits and he has developed one of the most extensive data bases on the subject.

Beutler writes clearly about the connection between EFA's and prostaglandins (powerful hormone-like substances which govern nearly every biologic function in our bodies), as well as about lignans (a phytochemical in flaxseed).

According to Beutler, giving attention to eating the omega-6's and the omega-3's in an overall healthy, balanced ratio (he suggests a 1:1 ratio) is important because prostaglandins are then also produced in a healthy and proper balance. A hitch can occur in this scenario, however. While omega-6 and omega-3 fatty acids are precursors in the production of prostaglandins, they actually compete with one another in these conversions. Furthermore, while certain prostaglandins can be a major ally in maintaining and rejuvenating health, other prostaglandins can, when out of balance with the others, seriously "gum up the works," contributing to a chemical chaos that can tear health to pieces. The health dividends for paying some attention to eating these fatty acids in a closer to healthy balance are enormous. (As I have already pointed out. Yet I roll my eyes to think about how rarely this is the case.)

In his article, "Fats for Health" (*Health Perspectives*, Mar/Apr. 1996, p.3) Beutler presents the following list of body systems and functions which depend on the proper quantity and balance of these EFAs.

Body Systems and Functions Dependent Upon EFAs:

- Steroid production and hormone synthesis
- Regulation of pressure in the eye, joints and blood vessels
- Regulation and response to pain, inflammation and swelling
- Mediation of immune response

- Regulation of bodily secretions and their viscosity
- Dilation or constriction of blood vessels
- Regulation of collateral circulation
- Direction of endocrine hormones to their target cells
- Regulation of smooth muscle and autonomic reflexes
- EFAs are primary constituents of cellular membranes
- Regulation of the rate at which cells divide (mitosis)
- EFAs maintain the fluidity and rigidity of cellular membrane
- EFAs regulates the in flow and out flux of substances into and out of the cells
- EFAs are important for transport of oxygen from the red blood cells to the bodily tissues
- Regulation of kidney function and fluid balance
- EFAs are important in keeping saturated fats mobile in the blood stream
- EFAs prevent blood cells from clumping together (the cause of atherosclerotic plaque and blood clots, a cause of stroke)
- Mediation of the release of pro-inflammatory substances from cells that may trigger allergic conditions
- EFAs serve as the primary energy source for the heart muscle
- Regulation of nerve transmission
- EFAs stimulate steroid production

Lignans Are It

Flaxseed contains a trace amount of vitamin E, along with beta carotene (pro-vitamin A), at least 23 trace minerals, and phytochemicals called *lignans*. Lignans are also present, but in lesser amounts, in other plant sources including vegetables and grains. Vitamin E and beta carotene, even in small amounts, act as antioxidants which enhance the functioning of the immune system and lessen damage to our cells from all sorts of toxins and pollutants. Lignans are significantly implicated in the prevention of serious disease such as heart disease and cancer.

Plant lignans in flaxseed oil are converted by bacteria in the human colon (actually in all mammals) to become mammalian lignans, which then bind with estrogen receptors to begin a chain of events thought to lessen the risk of developing certain types of cancer, especially breast and colon cancers. In 1993, in New Orleans, the FDA and the National Cancer Institute, as well as other research institutions, presented positive findings on the lignan-cancer connection at the annual convention on Experimental Biology.

Lignans are largely removed when flaxseed is pressed to obtain its oil; high concentrations of lignans remain in the flax pulp after pressing. Some state-of-the-art companies now produce a flaxseed oil with some of the pulp retained. The pulp in this "high-in-lignan" flaxseed oil adds a subtle, nutty flavor to the light buttery quality of the oil. This is the type I always use.

TASOLE:

"Flax oil? Are you saying eat flaxseed oil? That's the same as linseed oil isn't it? That smelly stuff I use as a wood finish in my wood shop? Got any better ideas?"

It was Donald talking. He and his wife Pat are two of the stubbornest people I know when it comes to trying anything new. Whenever this pair asks my opinion about how to improve their diets, they immediately have second thoughts.

"I'm not suggesting you should eat the linseed oil from your wood shop," I said, trying to remain calm. "When the oil of flaxseed is used for food, it is referred to as flaxseed oil. As a food oil it is delicate and has to be processed with great care. Because flaxseed oil easily gets rancid, it must be processed and stored properly. For non-edible uses, like in your wood shop, it is processed differently and it is always labeled as linseed oil."

"It says right on the linseed oil can not to eat it," Donald threw in, with his characteristic humor.

I ignored that remark and continued. "You asked me what would be the best oil to add to your diet didn't you? I thought you just told me your doctor said you needed more healthy oil—uncooked oil—in your diet, not oils in the form of cooked or fried foods. (Even their doctor knew she had to be quite specific or the next thing you know Pat and Donald would be swearing she'd told them to eat more fried chicken!)

"You're right; we asked," Donald agreed. "But, how can flax oil possibly taste good enough to eat? I thought you'd recommend olive oil or sesame oil."

"I wanted to give you my best idea first. Of course those other oils are great too, so if you'd rather go for them I won't bother explaining about the ... "

"I want to hear the flax idea," Pat chimed in before I completed my sentence. "I told the doctor my hormones were feeling 'off' again and my skin seemed to be drying up. Donald's liver was acting up too. The doctor talked to us about the need for proper fatty acids in our diet. Now that I'm thinking about it, she mentioned flaxseed oil too, but then I recalled that I had tasted some once and didn't like it at all. So I quickly forgot her suggestion."

Usually this is the type of situation that gets me so impatient I throw up my hands in frustration. Knowing how resistant Pat and Donald can be I don't know why I continued on, but I did—probably because I was in the mood for a challenge that day.

"Let's do an experiment," I suggested. "Next time I'm in town I'll bring over three different brands of flax oil for you to try on different foods. Use about two or three tablespoons a day and see if you like any brand better than another." (I knew which one of the flax oils always tasted the best to most people, but I also knew it was best not to say so until they had decided for themselves.)

About two weeks after I had given them the oils to try I visited Pat and Donald. They were having a snack at their kitchen table.

"So, what happened?" I asked.

Donald grinned. "One oil tasted wonderful, but the other two ruined my food altogether, and the cat's food too!"

"The cat?" I asked, as I looked around for it.

"The mangy-looking cat that has adopted us," explained Pat. "We put a little of each of the oils on our cat's food on different days. Most of the time the cat took a sniff and left right away. When we tried those particular oils too we agreed with the cat!"

It was just like Donald and Pat to try out this experiment on their cat; one of the reasons I liked them so much. I would have done the same thing. That cat was a scroungy-looking pet rescued from an unknown but obviously horrible situation. The cat's fur was dull and patchy and the cat was thin and sickly.

I looked back at Donald. "You're eating flax oil on your cottage cheese right now, aren't you? Those oils I gave you couldn't have all been that bad."

"That's what I was about to tell you," Donald was talking while he finished his cottage cheese. "Two did taste horrible, but *that* one," Donald pointed with his spoon to a bottle on the counter, "was so good I was sure it must be a different oil. The cat loved it too! The others we are now using out in the wood shop as wood finish."

"You picked the Barlean's brand, as I thought you would," I told them. "My all-time favorite!"

That wasn't the end to the experiment though. About a month later I saw Pat and Donald again.

"Still eating your flax oil every day?" I asked.

Pat looked up from her project as she said, "Wouldn't be without it. I'm having a noticeable improvement in my skin, and my hormones are certainly more balanced than they have been for a long time. Donald's energy level has improved and his liver-function test results from the doctor are definitely better."

Just then the cat wandered in. I couldn't believe my eyes! This animal was the same color as the old cat, but had beautiful, even luxuriant fur, and clear eyes.

"Did the other cat die?" I asked tentatively.

"I know it's hard to believe, but that's the same cat," Pat beamed. "I swear it's the flax oil we've been putting on her food. Before that we had tried other oils, veterinary medicines, special foods ... you name it. With all that, she still always looked like she was about to die. But since the flax oil experiment, ... well ..."

To summarize this flaxseed oil information in practical terms: you absolutely need EFA's for health and longevity and you need them in the right amount and balance. Keeping the *10 Essential Foods* prominent in your diet, limiting your intake of cooked or unhealthily processed fats and oils (ordinary store-bought vegetable oils, margarines of all sorts, spreadable "pretend butters," etc.) and processed foods, as well as by adding a daily intake of one to three tablespoons of properly processed flaxseed oil will help achieve this necessary balance.

SHOPPING FOR FLAXSEED OIL and OTHER FOOD SKILLS

All flax oil products are not created equal. First, only purchase *organic* flaxseed oil. Next, check the flavor, as this is a reliable indicator of proper processing, packaging or subsequent storage. (The big difference in quality of flax oils will become obvious if you ever have the misfortune to taste improperly processed or handled flax oil.)

Flax oil is a highly delicate oil, and like other edible oils can be seriously damaged with prolonged exposure to oxygen (air), heat or light. Improperly manufactured flax oil will commonly have a bitter taste and unpleasant aroma either of which, taste or aroma, can be so strong as to call paint lacquer to mind. A good flax oil has a very light flavor, reminiscent of butter, with a delicate aroma (if any), and no hint of rancidity or bitterness. If you ever purchase flax oil that turns out to fit this negative description you should certainly not eat it, as damaged flax oil can be worse for your health than eating no flax oil at all!

Flax oil can also be purchased in supplement form—with varying amounts of flax oil held in various sizes of gelatin "pearls." This packaging is said to preserve and protect the oils, but I say: Handle, refrigerate and store these "pearls" as carefully as you would the bulk flax oil. Even though I agree that in some cases, for reasons of convenience or flavor (yes, there is the rare person who, even when acquiring the best quality flax oil just doesn't take to the flavor, however mild) a flax oil supplement in gelatin pearls may be called for, I am still highly suspicious of the quality of the oil in these supplements. It doesn't hurt to cut one of these flax pearls open to give the oil the taste test. Then, if satisfied, store them in the refrigerator, no matter what the label says.

All edible oils should be carefully stored in an airtight container in a cool dark place, such as a refrigerator or cool cupboard; and the extremely delicate oils such as flax oil should always be stored in the refrigerator, or freezer. For instance, if you buy more flax oil than you can use in a couple of months, put the remainder in the freezer and thaw it out when you need it. (Freezing can prolong the shelflife from four months to one year.) And never buy flax oil from a store that did not keep it refrigerated at all times.

Since flax oil is heat sensitive, *never cook with it* as this would be worse than not eating it at all. Add flax oil to your food *after* it is prepared. While it is fine to put flax oil on warm foods, I would suggest not putting it on "steaming-hot" foods. (For cooking with oils, see the information in Healthy Additions below.)

I highly recommend dipping a hunk of fresh bread into flax oil mixed with herbs, using a sprinkling of flax oil on pasta (after the pasta is served), putting it on cottage cheese or plain yogurt (a mixture that is highly therapeutic and healing to the body), or mixing it together with olive oil in salad dressing.

I always buy a "high lignan" variety of organic flaxseed oil. The lignans are held in the form of a finely-grained, chocolate-brown, residue of pressed flaxseed that needs to be shaken up into the oil each time it is served. However, no matter how much you shake the bottle each time, when the oil is finally gone there is still some of this nutritous lignan residue left at the bottom. (You can feel the weight of it even if you can't see it through the opaque plastic container.) So, the question arises of what to do with this healthy residue.

Here is my "used-to-be secret" recipe for this residue. I take my kitchen scissors and cut off the top half of the plastic flax oil bottle in order to scoop out this priceless residue, which I use for making a special spread. I thoroughly mix this lignan residue with an equal amount of dark brown miso. I use a thin layer of this tasty spread on bread I intend for sandwiches, or I put a spoonful on my plate as a condiment and eat it in tiny bits with each mouthful of a whole grain or vegetable dish.

Miso is a Japanese food, a somewhat salty-flavored, fermented soybean paste, or soybean plus grain paste (such as rice or barley miso). If you buy an unpasteurized miso variety, as I do, in addition to its wonderful nutrition you reap the benefit of its lively enzymes. My favorite type, and the type I use for this flaxseed lignan/miso spread, is unpasteurized *Red Traditional Barley Miso*, from the Miso Master Company. This is the only company I know of that sells unpasteurized miso; and this brand is usually available at most health food stores. Pasteurized miso could also be used. But, pasteurized or not, be sure to get miso made from whole grains, not the varieties made from white rice (and possibly sweeteners), the so-called "sweet" or "mellow" misos.

Lalitha's One and Only Flax Oil Favorite

Even though I am sometimes warned not to suggest one particular brand of any product over another, I tend to completely ignore these warnings. In following this obstinate tendency, I would like to report that I have tasted many brands of flax oil—

many of them to my great and gagging regret. For me there is no longer a contest. *Barlean's Organic Flaxseed Oil* wins my gold star. The Barlean's company (actually the Barlean family), uses organic, scrupulously inspected flaxseed, presses their oil in small batches using an exclusive process partly inspired by Dr. Johanna Budwig and developed by the Barlean family, and ships directly to retail stores (using no middlemen) in order to shorten the time from press to consumer. Their flax oil is the "gold standard" by which I judge the quality of other oils; and yes, I am sure there must be other good ones out there for the educated consumer to find.

HEALTHY ADDITIONS, ALTERNATIVES, and TRAVELERS TIPS

While flaxseed oil is highly nutritious, it is what I call a "supplemental oil" which means that most people will want to have Additional healthy oils in their diet for other purposes, such as cooking. In fact, it is a good idea to eat 1 to 3 tablespoons of a variety of healthy oils, in addition to or including flax, each day.

The oils on the following list make good-tasting and healthy dietary Additions for variety; but there really is no overall Alternative—considering sources, availability, price and processing—for the omega-3 content of flaxseed oil itself.

I suggest that you try:

- *Extra Virgin Olive oil. Starred (*) oils can be found in an unrefined form at health food stores and are, therefore, the top choices.
- *Sesame oil:
- Almond oil
- Sunflower seed oil
- Pumpkin seed oil
- Avocado oil
- *Safflower oil (a good choice *only* if it is unrefined and organic. Spectrum Naturals brand has one that is refined and one that isn't, so read the labels.)

If you want to check out if an oil would be a good Addition to your diet, pay attention to the following criteria and try to find as many of these qualities as you can in the oils you choose. High-quality edible oils should be:

- Cold-pressed (best is mechanical expeller-pressed)

- Packaged in opaque (light-resistant) containers
- Unrefined, or refined with the most benign agents possible when refinement is necessary (these brands are usually found only in health stores)
- Organic where available

In addition to Barlean's brand, Spectrum Naturals and Hains are two other good brands of oils (available in health food stores and in some supermarkets), which often possess many of the above-mentioned qualities; but not in every case, so read the labels. The type of processing used with edible oils can make all the difference between "slow-death-with-fats-and-oils" and "profound-rejuvenation-with-fats-and-oils." For instance, you can buy highly-refined, non-organic safflower oil full of extreme contaminants and toxic refinements which contribute to a nasty interference in your health. Or, you can buy cold-pressed, unrefined, organic safflower oil and reap some health benefits. (Most generic grocery store brands of oils are of the "slow death" type.)

In my own home, I use flax oil and extra virgin olive oil almost exclusively. Extra virgin olive oil is a nutritious and healing food in its own right. Even though much can go wrong in the progress from seed to oil, olive oil, by its very nature, calls for little if any refining compared to most others. Whether or not you buy olive oil which is labeled *organic* or *unrefined*, if you buy cold-pressed extra virgin or virgin olive oil (as opposed to "pure" or "lite" which is polite talk for solvent-extraction methods), you will already have bypassed one of the steps involving major use of chemicals. After that, with extra virgin or virgin olive oil, only relatively minimal processing is done on it. Spectrum Naturals offers an unrefined olive oil.

Olive oil also has EFA's and is mostly fat of the mono-unsaturated (very healthy) type. Over and over I come across research proving olive oil to be a "longevity food" and a definitive help towards preventing heart disease. In one famous olive oil study reported in Jean Carper's book *Food Your Miracle Medicine*, Mediterranean peoples known for their high consumption of olive oil were found to have significantly less heart disease. In fact, the most enthusiastic consumers of olive oil were also the least likely to die of cancer or anything else! Of course the Mediterranean countries have access to the best-quality olive oil, and we can too, if we learn how to shop for it.

Olive oil can stand some heating without the unhealthy breakdown of its components, and should be the oil of choice if fried food is still desired, although fried foods in general should be highly limited. In any case, cooking-oil should not be allowed to get so hot that it smokes, as this signals the most serious and unhealthy breakdown of the oil's components.

The other oils listed above are strengthening and delightful foods, but they break down more readily when heat is applied, making them less healthy, or even harmful. Therefore, I don't use them for any type of cooking. (I won't be surprised if I get some arguments on this opinion from various oil experts because some oils are marketed as heat-tolerant for cooking—safflower oil or canola oil for example. These oils must be highly refined to be heat tolerant, however, although I do include them among my Survival Choices below.)

A Good Trick for Cooking With Oil

Whether you intend to "fry" some potatoes, sauté some onions or sizzle a steak, start off by heating a little water with added herbs, in the frying pan. Next add the items you would normally fry in oil or butter, and let them simmer. Then add a tablespoon or two of olive oil *as you cook*, while the extra water is steaming away. This lowers the cooking temperature that the oil is exposed to and often lessens the amount of cooking oil you need altogether.

SURVIVAL CHOICES for COMPROMISING CIRCUMSTANCES

For survival-level dietary oil choices in general, at least try to get cold-pressed oil. Try soy oil, safflower oil, or canola oil. Many people have touted these as healthy oils to be used copiously in the diet, and they are commonly available in supermarkets. I exclude them from my top choices for reasons of unacceptable levels of contamination with toxic chemicals such as pesticides, preservatives or solvents. Unless organically grown, the safflower plant, for example, is commonly sprayed with high amounts of chemicals while it is growing, as are many seed-oil plants. These contaminants become concentrated in the oil. However, the good news is that the oils on this list have a chance of being light years ahead in quality compared to the most common vegetable oil combinations usually seen on grocery store shelves. If you see something labeled *Vegetable Oil*, or *Cooking Oil*, don't even think about buying it.

At times you will find yourself in circumstances where you can't avoid eating cooked and unhealthy oils—they may be in various foods at restaurants, or served by your host where you are visiting. Or, you may find that whether the fats and oils are healthy or not you have a hard time digesting them. Whatever the case, you can help lessen the digestive stress and negative health effects in these situations with the use of a digestive enzyme supplement, especially the ones which contain the enzymes needed for the digestion of fats and oils. Your local health food stores will have several good choices for digestive enzymes. (See Supplies Appendix B.)

Survival Information for Margarine Users

For those who simply must have something thick and spreadable in place of butter, and have fallen for the false advertising that insists that margarines are good for you, here is the bad and the good news. (I say this even though I think you really should forget the spreadable idea and go for luscious flax oil or olive oil mixed with herbs and drizzled onto foods.)

Bad News

Hydrogenated fats or oils are found in abundance in margarine, baked goods, ready-made frostings and whips, frozen fish sticks, French fries, most fried fast-foods, imitation cheese, candies, etc. (Are you getting the picture?) Such items don't even make my Survival List because we won't survive very long or very well with them in our diets.

The hydrogenated and partially hydrogenated oils in margarines can increase "bad" cholesterol on a par with, or possibly worse than, animal fats such as butter! Margarines are shockingly high in the unhealthy trans-fatty acids (which are the result of an extremely nasty twisting of the molecules of the healthy fatty acids during hydrogenation).

When you take a fluid oil and try to make it stay thicker, you get hydrogenated or partially-hydrogenated oils, i.e., margarine, for one. A tub-type or squeeze-bottle margarine is less hydrogenated than the stick type, yet in all cases the damage is done. Any product (and there are probably thousands) that contains hydrogenated or partially hydrogenated oils is going to be feeding you these trans-fatty acids.

Trans-fatty acids are known to do the same types of harm to our bodies that unhealthy types of naturally saturated fats do.

(One way to observe saturated fats is that they are the ones that stay thick at room temperature, such as butter or the fat on a steak.) And, as I will soon point out, ounce for ounce butter proves to be at least an equal choice with margarine on the "poor choice" scale, or perhaps even a cut above, for those occasions when one simply cannot do without one or the other. The most commonly known harmful effects of eating trans-fatty acids are serious health difficulties such as heart disease, the raising of harmful LDL cholesterol, and the increased risk of immune-related diseases because of the harm the trans-fats do to the immune system (lowering B-cell response and causing T-cells to proliferate).

Here is what some of the news media have said on the subject of hydrogenation and trans-fatty acids:

San Francisco Chronicle   October 7, 1992
"Scientists Find Health Hazard In Margarine"
"A study by Dutch scientists, reported by the *New England Journal of Medicine* in 1990, was the first to cause widespread concern. It showed that trans-fatty acids raise levels of the harmful elements in cholesterol while lowering levels of the protective elements. The Agriculture Department [*USDA in 1992*] has now confirmed the Dutch study."

Los Angeles Times   March 4, 1993
"Beyond Trans-Fatty"
"...trans-fatty acids are as bad for your cholesterol as the saturated fats in butter. Now there's a trans-fatty acid free margarine—thickened with xanthan and guar gum rather than by hydrogenation..." [Spectrum Spread *from Spectrum Naturals is one such product; available at health stores.*]

Atlanta Journal   March 18, 1993
"Non-hydrogenated Oils Good on the Heart"
"You don't have to be a cardiologist to understand hydrogenation. The latest data indicates that even partially hydrogenated oils can cause heart disease."

San Francisco Chronicle   May 16, 1994
"Report Calls Margarine Deadly"
"An article being published today raises the possibility that margarine and other processed foods could be the cause of 30,000 of the nation's heart disease deaths ... A year ago,

researchers at the Harvard School of Public Health announced findings that margarine can increase the risk for heart disease in women by as much as 70 percent ... The article [*being published this day*] was written by Harvard nutritionist Walter Willett, renowned worldwide as one of the leading researchers on diet and heart disease. "Will people be shocked? I suspect so," Willett told the Associated Press ... In it, Willett poses the danger of what scientists have come to call trans-fats, which are produced during the hydrogenation process."

***

If you are one of the millions who have fallen for the "megabuck" margarine advertising, you have plenty of company. But, now that we are all more well informed, its time for a change.

The Good News

The good news is that public concern about hydrogenated and partially hydrogenated fats and oils has been piqued enough that the food industry is beginning to offer better products to the die-hard margarine users. Spectrum Naturals makes a product called *Spectrum Naturals Spread* that comes in a tub, has the consistency of most whipped spreads, has a buttery flavor, is not hydrogenated at all and is made from expeller-pressed canola oil. Spectrum Naturals company advertises that this product has no trans-fats, but warns that it should definitely not be used for cooking (as this would damage the fats; changing them into an unhealthy substance). This spread is still a highly processed product, however, and I don't suggest eating a lot of it. But, for those who need a survival choice while working up to my "first choice" list, you may want to give this spread a try

KIDS LOVE THIS

Spread a Brown Rice cake (a circular cracker about 1/2 inch thick made solely from puffed Brown Rice and found at most grocery stores in the cracker department) with a thin coating of raw, unfiltered honey. Next, drizzle on flaxseed oil. The result is a cracker that tastes like it is spread with butter and honey! This idea can work with any cracker, but children I work with like it best on the Rice cake. I do too. Many people like a cracker or bread, spread solely with *Barlean's Organic Flaxseed Oil.*

A few irresistible recipes:

ANY SALAD DRESSING

Using any salad dressing recipe, substitute 1/3 to 1/2 of the oil called for with flaxseed oil. The flaxseed oil mixes well with other oils, such as olive oil, while contributing to a heightened variety and amount of essential fatty acids.

SESAME SEED HONEY BALLS

1 cup raw unhulled sesame seeds
2 Tbs. flaxseed oil
2 Tbs. raw honey
1 Tbs. water

In a dry pan, heat/roast the sesame seeds until they begin to start popping, stirring occasionally to keep them from sticking. Still randomly stirring, let the seeds pop (roast) for 30 seconds to 1 minute and then take off the heat. They should be a very light-toasted cream-color, not dark-roasted. In a grinder or blender, blend the sesame seeds into a fine powder. Add all the other ingredients and mix into a smooth spread. Add more or less water, oil, or honey to adjust the consistency and sweetness for various tastes. Use as a vegetable dip, cracker spread, or just eat it on a spoon.

Recipes from: Lalitha's kitchen. (Note: The flavor of these recipes is based on using Barlean's flaxseed oil.)

CINNAMON-HONEY GRAPEFRUIT

1 whole fresh grapefruit (pink or white)
1/4 tsp. powdered cinnamon
1 1/2 tsp. raw honey
3 tsp. water

Cut the grapefruit in half. Cut around each section in each half of grapefruit so that each "bite" can be easily lifted.

Mix the honey and water together, then drizzle this honey-water onto each half of grapefruit. Sprinkle approximately one eighth teaspoon powdered cinnamon onto each half grapefruit— more or less to taste. Garnish with grated orange peel if desired.

Optional: Instead of cutting the grapefruit in half, peel and section the grapefruit, cutting each section into bite-size pieces and placing them in individual serving bowls. Drizzle on the honey-water and then sprinkle on the cinnamon. Garnish with grated orange peel if desired.

Recipe from: Lalitha's kitchen.

FUNCTIONAL COMPONENTS
In 100 Grams Raw Grapefruit
Serving Size: 1/2 to 2/3 fruit of one fresh raw grapefruit, approximately 100 grams, red, pink or white

Calories	32.0
Protein	1.0 g
Fat	.10 g
Carbohydrates	8.08 g
Fiber	.20 g
Cholesterol	0
Calcium	12.0 mg
Phosphorus	8.0 mg
Magnesium	8.0 mg
Potassium	139.0 mg
Sodium	0
Iron	.09 mg
Copper	.047 mg
Manganese	.012 mg
Zinc	.07 mg
Selenium	trace
Chromium	trace
Vitamin A	124.0 mg
Vitamin C	37.0 mg
Vitamin B1 (Thiamin)	.036 mg
Vitamin B2 (Riboflavin)	.020 mg
Vitamin B3 (Niacin)	.250 mg
Vitamin B6	.042 mg
Folacin	10.2 mcg
Vitamin 12	0
Pantothenic Acid (Vit. B5)	.283 mg
Vitamin E	0
Biotin	1.8 mcg

Prominent Phytochemicals and Antioxidants in Grapefruit:
Beta-carotene, lycopene (these first two are found in significantly higher amounts in the red and pink grapefruits), quercetin, courmarins, galacturonic acid, citrus pectin, vitamin C

Sources:
1) Santillo, Humbart, N.D. *Intuitive Eating* (Prescott, AZ: Hohm Press, 1993).
2) Margen, Sheldon, M.D. and the Editors of the University of California at Berkeley "Wellness Newsletter." *The Wellness Encyclopedia of Food and Nutrition* (New York, NY: Rebus Press [Random House], 1992).

10

GRAPEFRUIT

WHAT IS SO GOOD ABOUT GRAPEFRUIT?

I take grapefruit quite seriously. Pink or Ruby grapefruit are my all-time favorites for flavor and nutritional content, although my father grows some of the sweetest "yellow" grapefruit around, outside his Phoenix home. I love it when he brings some of these juicy beauties over to my house.

Working together, the functional components of the whole inner pulp of grapefruit (by the way, the red and pink varieties are the most potent in several functional components) give it the well-deserved reputation for:

- lowering cholesterol
- anti-cancer activity (particularly against stomach and pancreatic cancers)
- enhancing the immune system
- building alkaline mineral reserves
- anti-viral activity
- anti-bacterial activity
- protecting arteries
- enhancing health of the cardiovascular system
- stimulating digestion

In Jean Carper's *Food Your Miracle Medicine* (p. 210) (see Recommended Bibliography), she describes citrus research by toxicologist Herbert Pierson, Ph.D., a diet and cancer expert formerly with the National Cancer Institute. Pierson calls citrus fruits a total anticancer package, because they possess every class of natural substances (carotenoids, flavonoids, terpenes, limonoids, and coumarins) that individually have neutralized powerful chemical carcinogens in animals. One analysis found that citrus fruits possess fifty-eight known anticancer chemicals; more than any other food.

The Pulp Is It!

Before I get into the details of the functional components in grapefruit, I would like to set a clear groundrule about this important food. It is a mistake to think that you can get all the wonderful benefits of having grapefruit in your diet by solely drinking grapefruit juice, even if it is freshly pressed and delicious. Those fine white membranes that separate each section of the inner pulp, the spongy white inner lining of the peel, and even the seeds, are indispensable carriers of health-maintaining substances that, along with the inner pulp of each section (juice held in those tiny juice sacs/membranes), offer an irreplaceable package of phytochemicals, fiber, flavor and nutrition.

It is not necessary to eat all the peels and seeds of every grapefruit one ingests in order to make good out of it. I am suggesting the moderate approach of simply eating the delicate membranous parts of the inner sections of a half or whole grapefruit. This, along with inventing various toppings for the less sweet types of grapefruits, may be all one ever wants to do. (By the way, my favorite "grapefruit-drizzle" topping is raw honey mixed with enough water to make it drizzle properly.)

I also like to go a little further with my grapefruit adventure and take a nip of the white, spongy inner side of the peel and eat a seed or two for the powerful benefits offered there. Of course I keep grapefruit juice on my dietary repertoire because I truly enjoy it, and grapefruit juice still has highly desirable qualities. In fact, I often use freshly-squeezed grapefruit juice as a major ingredient in my salad dressing instead of most of the vinegar.

Eating a few grapefruits seeds is not just a silly idea of Lalitha's. As you can imagine, the seed of a plant holds the detonating force of creation. Philosophically speaking, therefore, you may agree that this mysterious power-packed tidbit (seed) might enhance your life in highly desirable, even if unknown, ways. However, you may not yet be aware of how wide-ranging this enhancement can be.

A powerful healing substance made from the seeds and juiceless pulp of grapefruit is now marketed. This grapefruit pulp and seed concentrate is available in an almost-clear liquid form, having the consistency of honey, or as tablets or capsules. Bio/Chem Research Inc., one of the foremost manufacturers of the basic material (*Citricidal®*) used in many standardized grapefruit extract products claims:

> Grapefruit extract is manufactured via a unique bio-technical process that isolates all the natural protective elements from the seeds and pulp of the fruit. This natural grapefruit extract has been shown effective against over 100 micro-organisms [pathogens/germs] including:
> —Gram-positive bacteria such as Staphylococcus, Streptococcus and Listeria.
> —Gram-negative bacteria such as E.Coli, Klebsiella, Legionella, Salmonella, Shigella, Cholera and Pseudomonas.
> —Fungi and Yeasts such as Candida, Aspergillus and Trichophyton.
> —Viruses such as Herpes simplex 1, Influenza A2, and some animal viruses.
> —Parasites such as Giardia lamblia, Entamoeba histolytica and Chlamydia.

This is an impressive list, and I have much experience to prove that this list is not exaggerated, whether I am using the extract, or an herbal poultice of the whole grapefruit pulp, depending on the situation. My friends and I have used the extract (my favorite sources are NutriBiotic® and Allergy Research Inc. brands, (available at health stores), for colds and flu; as a douche for many types of vaginal infections including yeast; for traveler's diarrhea; for ear-nose-mouth infections, and much more. One of the most frequent jobs I use grapefruit extract for is in disinfecting foods after bringing them home from the store. (I give detailed instructions about this "disinfecting detox-soak" in chapter 2.) For an authoritative and practical resource on the many uses of this powerful and effective substance see: *The Healing Power of Grapefruit Seed* (Sharamon, Sheila and Baginski, Bodo J., Twin Lakes, WI: Lotus Light Publications, 1996. 1-800-548-3824).

What all this has to do with me eating a couple of grapefruit seeds is that I know it is smart to be eating the whole food from which this extract is made. I know that phytochemicals are strong and that only tiny amounts are needed to have a positive cumulative effect, even the tiny amount found in a single grapefruit seed. So, I eat the whole grapefruit on a regular basis, including some seeds, and if I get in a situation where I need an extra potent concentrate without the nasty side effects and inefficiencies of allopathic medicines (which is almost always), I use the grapefruit extract. In fact, I never travel without it.

MAJOR FUNCTIONAL COMPONENTS

Among the major functional components found in the whole inner pulp and membranes of grapefruit, I have chosen to focus on vitamin C, the phytochemicals: beta-carotene, lycopene, quercetin, coumarins and galacturonic acid (a type of soluble fiber); citrus pectin; and a whole cascade of vital minerals.

Grapefruit, as well as all citrus, is commonly known as a significant source of vitamin C which enhances the body's immune system, lessens the effects of stress, helps prevent heart disease, lessens or prevents symptoms of colds and flu, has anticancer properties and numerous other health benefits. A good deal of this vitamin C is in the fresh juice of the citrus, in this case the grapefruit.

The hearty amounts and the variety of major minerals in a serving of grapefruit (see the listing at the beginning of the chapter) contribute to the smooth working of every single function in the body and help buffer the mild natural acids that are also present in the grapefruit. (That's one of the reasons that I chose grapefruit over, say, lemon in the group of citrus as one of my "Top 10" foods. Although lemon is a potent healing food which I often use for medicinal purposes, the acid and mineral ratio in lemon makes it too acidic for most people to eat pleasurably on a regular basis as a whole food. Whereas grapefruit, with its many varieties, is enjoyable in some form for almost everyone.)

Dr. Humbart "Smokey" Santillo, in his book *Intuitive Eating* (p. 83), mentions an interesting fact about the interplay of the acids and minerals in grapefruit (and citrus in general). After discussing how minerals are important for buffering acids in our body fluids, he goes on to say:

> Although these foods [*citrus*] have organic acids
> in them, these mild acids are cleansing to the

system, are oxidized into CO_2 and water, and do not create an [*unhealthy*] acid effect on the body fluids. They also contain high concentrations of [*health-promoting*] alkaline minerals which, after digestion, increase the body's alkaline mineral reserves.

Dr. Santillo also points out that much citrus is grown on depleted soils which adversely affect the acid and mineral balance of the fruit. Keeping this in mind, I once again suggest the use of organic foods.

TASOLE:

"I thought I would love eating rich French food, and as much as I wanted every day; but my body is just not agreeing with my mind."

I overheard this part of a conversation between two of my ten traveling companions as we jostled along yet another winding road in the French countryside. In this case, Nancy was speaking to Richard, but several others threw in comments of agreement. This was day number three of a sixteen-day trip, and we all knew the trip would involve many more of these jostling, rented-van-on-a-winding-road excursions to meet the people we had come to see ... as they all lived in out-of-the-way places.

We were all friends, traveling together for business, but the pleasure aspect was admittedly not far behind in priority. We passed from one host's hands to the next and were treated royally, especially in the food department.

"I love the flavors and textures of the food!" Nancy continued, "I'm beginning to worry that each host is becoming more flamboyant than the last in the way they are feeding us. I'm still stuffed after a wonderful breakfast and then ... there comes lunch. But ooohh, I can't stop myself. The food here is all so attractive."

I was also feeling a little overdone by the sheer amount of rich food with exotic sauces when Richard spoke up. "I think it would be rude to not eat what a host was offering, but it certainly gets my stomach churned up when we have to go from one of those feasts back into this van for a roller-coaster ride the rest of the day." At this point, Richard, whose sense of humor I only sometimes appreciate, grabbed exaggeratedly for one of the car-sickness bags. His mock "gagging" sounds were accompanied by spastic thrashings about, his eyes bulging comically. That Richard!

Two less dramatic companions, who I knew were also suffering from what I call "liver headaches," simply tried to sleep through the pain on the way to the next meal. Since this was only the third day and I wanted to survive in good form, I immediately decided to try something a Japanese healer friend had taught me long ago.

"Always eat at least half a grapefruit after a rich meal, or while traveling and eating foods one is not used to," the healer had wisely advised. When we stopped near a market I slipped off to buy myself a grapefruit so I would be ready after the next meal.

"How can you still be eating anything after that huge meal?" Nancy had noticed me, after our meal, sitting in the van, munching on slices peeled from half a grapefruit. I offered her some. "I couldn't hold another thing," she protested.

I tried to explain, a little. "My Japanese healer friend told me about this trick. Eating a sour food (and I don't mean lemon drop candies, I admonished her), such as citrus and especially grapefruit, before and/or after a heavy or rich meal, helps stimulate the liver's digestive output so it doesn't become congested. The citrus also adds a healthy dose of much needed alkaline minerals to the digestive process, along with organic acids which are gently cleansing. He said it could settle an over-stuffed stomach, and encourage food to move through quickly."

"He must have loved his grapefruit," Nancy said with a laugh. "I've never thought that much about grapefruit myself."

I continued on a bit more. "One of the main points of interest to me right now is that he said this idea was particularly useful after eating foods containing fats, oils, cream, etc., or simply after eating too much food on occasion. Sure you don't want some?"

Nancy sat down and ate a few grapefruit slices with me. Then it was time to go to a meeting where normally several of us would be struggling, me included, to stay awake following our rich meal. This evening, however, Nancy and I both stayed alert.

"I don't have the usual headache. I wasn't so sleepy and my last meal isn't feeling like it wants to take up permanent residence. Maybe I'm getting used to the food, do you think?" Nancy offered enthusiastically.

"It could be the grapefruit, because I'm feeling the same way," I said. "I'm off to buy another grapefruit for after dinner tonight; so I'll see you at the next meeting."

After dinner that evening, sure enough Nancy "happened" to stroll by where I was sitting peeling my grapefruit.

"Do you want to split that grapefruit? It looks too big for one person," Nancy asked. "You know what my Chinese grandmother always says about French grapefruit ..." (She had no Chinese grandmother, of course. She was playfully teasing me.) "Besides," Nancy added with a wink, "isn't it supposed to be bad luck to eat one of those big honkers by yourself?"(Translation: "honker" [in English or French] means something is extra large).

I gave Nancy a half, and after we ate it we stayed up a while talking with a few of the others before going to bed. Right before we walked off to our rooms, Sandra showed up. "I'm not used to eating rich food three times a day. I think that's why I'm getting a headache now after some meals. How are you two feeling?" she asked us.

Nancy and I smiled at each other as we answered, in chorus, "Great!"

"Have you been at all the meals?" Sandra asked. "Even Richard, who has a huge capacity and total tolerance for any type of food, is slowing down."

Nancy told Sandra about the grapefruit trick and then we all went off to sleep. The next morning I was peeling my grapefruit when Sandra showed up with one of her own and sat down next to me. Then, Nancy showed up, looking longingly at our grapefruits. I reached for the second one I had bought in case of such emergencies and handed it to her. "All right! All right! I'll start buying my own grapefruit; but for now, give me that!" and she jokingly dove for the spare fruit.

The next day ... and the next, our schedule was so tight we did not have an opportunity to buy grapefruit. Sharon, Nancy and I each noticed an unpleasant difference without them. On the third day, however, I had gotten a grapefruit from the cook where we were staying and had taken it along with me in the van, thinking to peel it as we rode along. It was far too juicy and I had no napkins, so I decided to wait and discreetly eat it at the next rest stop.

There I was, hunkered down between two trees in the French countryside, trying to get out of the ferocious wind and with grapefruit juice streaming down my hands and face, thinking I was all alone for the moment. One by one my companions walked up and squatted down around me just starring at my only grapefruit like it was the last piece of food on earth. The word had spread! Everyone wanted a piece of the "grapefruit action." Apparently Richard had questioned Nancy and Sandra about why we were eating grapefruit, and then Richard had talked to Debbie, and on and on.

"OK," I said, "you each get one slice; but we're stocking up at the next store!" They all agreed.

Among the circle of our business associates it didn't take long for "those Americans" to get a reputation for having a grapefruit fetish. But the French, being the superb hosts that they are, soon began to offer grapefruit to us everywhere we went.

(The story ends here, but in all fairness I must add that, over the years, I have ocassionally discovered a friend for whom this "eating grapefruit after a meal" trick is a poor food combination resulting in intestinal gas. Each must decide for oneself!)

The benefits of beta carotene are covered in the chapter on Carrots, so I'll quickly recap here. Beta carotene is a phytochemical that is metabolized in the liver into vitamin A, and is often referred to as "pro-vitamin A." It is an antioxidant associated with anti-aging, healthy body tissues, anticancer activity, help with PMS, asthma, ulcers and acne, as well as general immune system enhancement.

The red and pink varieties of grapefruit are significantly higher in beta carotene than the light yellow varieties. Among the *10 Essential Foods*, although pink and red grapefruit are no slouches in the beta carotene department, Carrots and Spinach are even higher yet. (You'll have no lack of opportunities for getting a good daily dose of this rejuvenating phytochemical when using the *10 Essential Foods*, because all of them contain beta carotene to some degree!)

Coumarins are a class of phytochemicals found in high amounts in tomatoes and citrus fruits such as grapefruit. As with many phytochemicals being studied, coumarins are showing anticancer activity. In addition, coumarins show activity for help with inflammation, fungus infection and immune stimulation.

Quercetin, one of many flavonoids found in grapefruit, is present in particularly generous amounts. I have used quercetin as a supplement, along with my regular grapefruit, especially during hayfever season—since quercetin has noticeable antihistamine action. Sometimes, just eating an extra bit of the white part of the grapefruit helps my hayfever. According to the USDA database on phytochemicals, quercetin shows a long list of "anti" activities—antihistimine, antiviral, anti-asthmatic, antileukemic, antimalarial, and antioxidant, to name a few!

You can get noticeable quercetin help by simply eating grapefruit. If you already have bothersome symptoms of some of the health concerns I just listed, you can always buy an extra quercetin supplement to go along with your grapefruit. (Don't just use the quercetin supplement, leaving out the grapefruit. All sorts of other functional components in the grapefruit enhance the action of quercetin. You just can't get that degree of help with the isolated quercetin in a tablet.)

Galacturonic acid, a special type of fiber found in grapefruits, has cholesterol-lowering activity. (You've got to eat the whole segments, though, not just drink grapefruit juice. The juice does not contain the galacturonic acid.) A study by Dr. James Cerda of the University of Florida showed that when subjects ate about two and a half cups of grapefruit segments every day, they lowered their cholesterol by about 10 %

Citrus pectin is a water-soluble fiber found in the pulp of grapefruit and other citrus fruits. Julian Whitaker, M.D. describes its cancer-fighting potential (*Health and Healing*, May 1966, p. 6):

> If you've ever made jam or jelly, most likely you used pectin to set the mixture. In a special process, the citrus pectin is "modified" or broken down into particles small enough to be absorbed into the bloodstream. [*Lalitha believes this also happens in digestive processes.*] There it binds to tumor cells and interferes with their adherence to receptor cells in secondary sites in the body, thus preventing metastasis. It's been called "cellular teflon" because it prevents cancer cells from adhering to anything. Animal studies have shown very positive results and although I am unaware of any human studies

204   10 ESSENTIAL FOODS

with pectin, I personally would add it to my
cancer-fighting arsenal. It's nontoxic, has no side
effects, and early research is very promising.
The recommended dose of modified citrus
pectin is one to two heaping teaspoons of powder (13 grams) in water per day. [See Citrus
Pectin in Supplies Appendix B.]

Citrus pectin from eating whole grapefruit is not as concentrated as the therapeutic doses recommended by Dr. Whitaker,
but it certainly adds some health benefit; and I for one like
knowing it is in each bite of grapefruit I eat!

Lycopene is a phytochemical from the carotene (carotenoid)
group, as is beta-carotene. Lycopene shows such important
antioxidant activity that some supplement manufacturers are
now marketing specific lycopene supplements (as they are
doing with quercetin and beta-carotene). Researchers at Johns
Hopkins University studied the blood of 26,000 people and
found that: "those with the least blood lycopene had over five
times the risk of pancreatic cancer as healthy people with the
most blood lycopene." (Carper, Jean. *Food Your Miracle
Medicine*, p. 257.) In addition to pink or red grapefruit, tomatoes
are another top source of lycopene.

Whenever I read about these studies of phytochemicals that
have anticancer activity (and there are many phytochemicals
and many studies in this regard) I can't help but speculate that
if an antioxidant substance such as lycopene is doing something to help prevent or reverse a serious disease like pancreatic cancer, it must also be positively and powerfully affecting
immune responses on a much broader scale. Such immune
strengthening assuredly helps prevent many other types of illnesses that may take hold when the body lacks the antioxidant
potential available in whole foods. And speaking of antioxidant
potential, grapefruit rates high.

Even though some phytochemicals have been isolated and
partially researched, there are still many hundreds that haven't
been looked into yet. It is becoming increasingly clear to science, as it has been to folk healers for ages, that it is the *combinations* of functional components that greatly enhance the activity of all of them. For example, carotenes are somewhat tissue-
specific (i.e., lycopene is especially protective of pancreatic tissue), and when several carotenes are present together (which is
the case with many whole, fresh foods), the broad spectrum
antioxidant activity is much greater than from a single

carotene. For example, pink or red grapefruit have lycopene and beta-carotene of the carotene group, and probably more.

If you consider the potential health benefits of this mix of carotenes in grapefruit, together with the unique activities of all the other functional components I've mentioned; if you then further contemplate the known and unknown ways these phytochemicals might enhance each other, you might just find yourself rushing out to your nearest grocery store, heading for the grapefruit bins!

SHOPPING FOR GRAPEFRUIT and OTHER FOOD SKILLS

Unlike much of the fruit at a grocery store, grapefruit is harvested fully ripe. This means that it has been given its full opportunity to completely develop the most dynamic maturity of its functional components. Of course, a lot depends on the richness of the soil it was grown in, so once again I suggest organic sources.

The grapefruit you pick out should be uniformly firm with none of those sick-feeling mushy spots that often occur from bruising when the citrus has been piled high in the store or abused during its handling. (Lots of my friends thought those soft areas were the normal thing, yet always wondered why the grapefruit they chose was often pithy, tasteless, or easily rotted.) Be finicky. Squeeze each grapefruit you are considering. If you are considering one of those bargain bags of grapefruit, look through the plastic and "eyeball" the fruit seriously, gently squeezing each one for firmness. I always hate it if I haven't done the grapefruit-squeeze test and then end up with a "lemon" in the bag which starts spoiling quickly when I get home.

Once you get hooked on eating grapefruit, you may develop a special ritual for eating it, like my friend Paul has. After a meal, he carefully peels a grapefruit, setting the peels aside. Then he takes each section, peels the membrane off of it, and pops the juicy middle parts into his mouth. Finally, he eats up all the membranes he has carefully saved and throws away the heavy outer peels. I haven't actually watched him that closely, but I seriously suspect that, like me, Paul regularly eats a couple of seeds. A wonderful side effect of the ritual is that his young children are now developing the grapefruit habit and regularly join him in eating a section of grapefruit after a meal. The youngest child always asks to have her section peeled of its membrane, but his five-year-old insists on doing his own, eating the membranes just like his dad.

HEALTHY ADDITIONS, ALTERNATIVES and TRAVELERS TIPS

To varying degrees, all citrus have similar qualities to grapefruit. And, all types of citrus, if eaten whole, certainly qualify for a healthy food choice. If I had to choose an Alternative to grapefruit I would probably take a lemon, and just eat less of it. (Of course I probably would put some honey-drizzle on it, although I do have friends who are crazy-in-love with eating lemons anytime and any place.) Realizing that I have been adamant about eating citrus whole, I will nevertheless state that lemon juice has long been used as a cleansing and healing food in alternative medicine circles. At restaurants I regularly ask for slices of lemon to squeeze into the pure water I order, for a great on-the-spot liver and digestive aid. This is one situation where the juice is all that is needed. (See the Lemon Body-Tonic in Guideline 9 of chapter 2.)

Oranges are excellent Additions if it means eating a whole, fresh orange now and then. Most people, however, overdo it with large amounts of orange juice. In my experience with hundreds of friends and students over the years, too much orange juice easily creates health difficulties—such as head congestion (especially in children), and extreme blood sugar fluctuations which, in the long run, adversely affect energy, mood, digestion and general health. The high amount of natural sugars, among other things in orange juice, is the probable cause. In addition, many folks (young and old) guzzle products called "orange drinks" that are really pasteurized, processed, watered down, flavored, junky substitutes for the real thing. So, for me, eating a whole fresh orange now and then supports the *10 Essential Foods* approach, but is not a substitute for grapefruit, or even lemon. Tangerines are another smart Addition.

SURVIVAL CHOICE for COMPROMISING SITUATIONS

Frozen grapefruit juice is my Survival Choice. If I am drinking packaged juice of any kind, in general I go for the frozen variety.

Using juices for mixed drinks, punches, snacks, etc., is perfectly fine as long as it doesn't replace eating whole citrus, especially when it is in season. Also, the Crystal Geyser company makes a delightful unsweetened and carbonated drink called

Grapefruit Juice Squeeze (usually a health store item) that I use now and then. Either frozen juice or this Crystal Geyser product would be better than most juice drinks from a can, bottle or carton, as these latter are more highly processed and often full of sugar, chemicals, flavoring, colorings and preservatives.

Another Survival trick, especially if you are in a hurry, is to squeeze a fresh grapefruit and drink the juice. Even if you don't eat the whole grapefruit, you still get nutritional benefit, immensely more than store-bought juice, and certainly better than no grapefruit at all. (I pop a seed or two into my mouth, for good measure. And yes, I *chew* them up regardless of how big a hurry I'm in.) I don't recommend getting yourself into a situation where you have to rush around like this, but I know we all do it.

While traveling in India and Mexico, particularly during the hot seasons, I would go to the open-air markets every day and buy whatever fresh citrus I could find. Usually it was some type of orange or tangerine, and occasionally I would eat some lemon. I would peel and eat these throughout the day and this saved me from dehydration even when I couldn't get safe water or safe food anywhere else. Plus, I reaped the benefits of the nutrition of the citrus. (I survived quite well; felt great in fact, even if this went on for days with only eating a plate of rice now and then.)

KIDS LOVE THIS

Pink or red grapefruit, eaten plain as these are the sweetest varieties, are a great hit with kids. Also, children enjoy sitting around a bowl of grapefruit segments which they can dip into another bowl containing "honey-drizzle," before popping the slice into their mouths.

Honey-drizzle is simply raw, unheated honey mixed with enough pure water to get a thin consistency for dipping. If you use straight honey, it is so thick that the honey is eaten in far too great a quantity for good health. The honey-drizzle is supposed to be thin enough to leave only a very light coating of sweet flavor.

Other healthy yet sweet syrups from the health food store, such as rice bran syrup, molasses, or barley malt could be made into creative drizzles, when drizzles are called for. But remember, lots of children like their pink grapefruit plain, and this is the best choice for regular use.

Unforgettable grapefruit treats:

CITRUS SALAD

Fresh citrus such as:
  grapefruit
  tangerine
  orange
  tangelo
  lemon

Peel, section, and cut into bite-size pieces various types of citrus (predominantly grapefruit), such as white grapefruit, pink grapefruit, tangerines, oranges and tangelos. Fill a bowl with the amount required of the citrus mixture (about 2/3 cup is a good individual serving).

As a dressing for this salad use raw honey, barley malt, or rice bran syrup mixed half and half with water, or use some of the citrus juice accumulating in the bottom of the citrus salad bowl instead of the water. Or, use undiluted grade A maple syrup.

Optional: To this mixture add shredded coconut and/or raisins to taste. A nice touch for lemon-lovers is to add a small amount of lemon cut into tinier-than-bite-size pieces.

SUMMER MAPLE GRAPEFRUIT

1 whole grapefruit (any color)
1/4 cup grade A Maple Syrup
1/4 cup grated, fresh or dried coconut
30 toothpicks (approximately)

Peel and section the grapefruit. Put a toothpick into each section of grapefruit and freeze the sections.

Using the toothpick as a holder, dip a frozen section of grapefruit into the maple syrup and then into the coconut. Eat!

Recipes from: Lalitha's kitchen

LOW-FAT SPINACH LASAGNA (serves 6)

1 10-ounce package frozen chopped spinach
1 to 2 Tbs. olive oil
1 1/2 to 2 cups chopped mushrooms
1 medium onion, chopped
1 pound of 1% cottage cheese
1/4 cup grated parmesan cheese
1 2/3 cups tomato sauce
9 lasagna noodles, cooked

Cook the spinach, squeeze out the excess moisture and set it aside.

Saute the onions and mushrooms in the olive oil until the onions are transparent and the mushrooms are cooked. When they have cooled slightly, mix in all of the cottage cheese and 2 tablespoons of the parmesan.

Layer in an 8 1/2" x 13" pan:
1/2 to 2/3 cup tomato sauce
3 cooked noodles. (Break the ends off so they will fit.)
all of the cooked spinach, spreading it out evenly
1/2 of the cheese/mushroom mixture
1/3 cup tomato sauce
3 more noodles
the rest of the cheese/mushroom mixture
3 more noodles
2/3 cup tomato sauce
2 Tbs. parmesan

Cover the pan [perhaps with a non-aluminum cookie sheet] and bake for 1/2 hour at 350°.

Lower the heat to 200° and bake another 1/2 hour uncovered, then put it under the broiler for a couple of minutes to lightly brown the top. It will cave in, but will taste great.

It freezes well. Make it ahead, then re-heat it. (Put the frozen lasagna in the oven at 250° for about an hour.) It gets better when it is re-heated once or even twice.

FUNCTIONAL COMPONENTS
In 100 Grams Raw Spinach
Serving Size: 1 cup, 55 grams, fresh raw spinach

Calories	220
Protein	3.0 g
Fat	.35 g
Carbohydrates	4.0 g
Fiber	.89 g
Cholesterol	0
Calcium	99.0 mg
Phosphorus	49.0 mg
Magnesium	79.0 mg
Potassium	558.0 mg
Sodium	79.0 mg
Iron	3.0 mg
Copper	.13 mg
Manganese	.90 mg
Zinc	.53 mg
Selenium	yes
Chromium	11.0 mcg
Vitamin A	7000.0 mcg
Vitamin C	28.0 mg
Vitamin B1 (Thiamin)	.078 mg
Vitamin B2 (Riboflavin)	.189 mg
Vitamin B3 (Niacin)	.724 mg
Vitamin B6	.195 mg
Folacin	100.0 mcg
Vitamin 12	0
Pantothenic Acid (Vit. B5)	.065 mg
Vitamin E	1.25 mg
Vitamin K	yes
Biotin	3.5 mcg

Prominent Phytochemicals and Antioxidants in Spinach:
Chlorophyll, lutein, zeaxanthin, beta carotene

Sources:
1) Santillo, Humbart, N.D. *Intuitive Eating* (Prescott, AZ: Hohm Press, 1993).
2) *Nutrition Almanac*, Nutrition Research, Inc. McGraw-Hill, 1984. Nutritional data used with permission of the McGraw-Hill companies.
3) Margen, Sheldon, M.D. and the Editors of the University of California at Berkeley "Wellness Newsletter." *The Wellness Encyclopedia of Food and Nutrition* (New York, NY: Rebus Press [Random House], 1992).

Recipe from: © Carol Anne Nostrand Johns, June 1996. Previously unpublished. Used with permission.

11

SPINACH

WHAT IS SO GOOD ABOUT SPINACH?

Green is Great!

Green foods get me excited! Two outstanding varieties amongst many in the heap of dark green foods are spinach and Sprouts. Whatever I tell you in this chapter about the priceless magic of green in spinach, will also apply in the next chapter to green leafy Sprouts. So, pay careful attention here so when you get to the Sprout chapter you'll be up to speed.

My green excitement is about chlorophyll, a unique substance in plants that works directly with the energy of the sun to convert that sun energy, through photosynthesis, into all the substances necessary to sustain life for the plant, while also giving plants their green color. Intriguingly, chlorophyll itself can *only* be made when sunlight is present! Lois Mattox Miller, writing for the *Science News Letter* over fifty-five years ago (March 15, 1941), poignantly described this amazing mystery/process of photosynthesis:

> A ray of sunlight strikes the green leaf and instantly the miracle is wrought. Within the plant, molecules of water and carbon dioxide are torn apart—a feat which the chemist can

accomplish only with great difficulty and expense. First there are only lifeless gas and water; then presto! These elements are transformed into living tissue and useful energy. Oxygen is released from the plant to revitalize the air we breathe. Units of energy, in sugars and other carbohydrates, are speedily manufactured and stored in the living plant.

I bet you knew chlorophyll was responsible for the green color of plants, and you also may have known that chlorophyll makes the crucial link with sunlight to sustain plant life, but did you know of its miraculous health-building and health-repairing qualities that extend to the animal kingdom, including humans?

I am not exaggerating. I have personally witnessed several miracles of chlorophyll and its "sister components," when used both internally and externally. For example, there was Bob who had what doctors kept telling him was "plain old tired blood." (Don't you just want to scream when you pay $80 a whack for three visits to the doctor and the verdict is that "your blood is 'tired'... and why don't you just take a nap and swallow a few vitamins that will only make you burp up nasty flavors ..."; yet you are still tired?) When Bob started adding dark green leafy foods like spinach, kale, Sprouts, and Swiss chard (no, iceberg lettuce does not count) to his diet every day he noticed a dramatic improvement. When he went even further and added a "green drink" (see the TASOLE below) at least every other day ... Wow! He perked up like a striped bass jumping for a fly on a sunny day. In the case of my friend Patricia who had persistent troubles with hemorrhoids and varicose veins, "eating green" induced a noticeable improvement within a week. Another friend, Sean, was a high performance athlete who, along with several companions, increased his stamina, concentration and performance quite significantly just by adding fresh greens to his daily diet, and in some cases taking an additional chlorophyll supplement.

In his book, *Chlorophyll Magic From Living Plant Life* (Escondido, CA: 1981), Dr. Bernard Jensen, chiropractor, nutritionist, health researcher, and "healer *extraordinaire*" describes case after case of health rejuvenation using chlorophyll. One memorable case history, which reminds me of many I have seen myself, involved a young woman with thirteen leg ulcers that had not healed in three years. Of course she had seen many doctors and been to several clinics. With Dr. Jensen's treatment this young woman's leg ulcers completely disappeared in three weeks. She simply drank three or four quarts each day of what Jensen called "chlorophyll-water." (He made this by chopping up nine different types of greens. Then he "left them for an hour or two in distilled water and then squeezed them through cheesecloth for her to drink.") Her "before and after" photographs are startling; yet, in my experience, not surprising at all. Dr. Jensen describes using chlorophyll plants as a general blood tonic and for helping everything from liver concerns, to ulcers, menstruation and hepatitis.

If you are starting off with generally good health, the rejuvenating and stamina-building potential you could easily reap by adding the *10 Essential Foods* "greens"—Spinach, Sprouts, and Broccoli — to your diet is virtually unlimited.

The Mysterious Green-ness

Science does not yet explain all the whys and wherefores of how chlorophyll works for our benefit (which makes me love it all the more). However, there are some "knowns" that will encourage even the most doubtful with the idea of "eating green." The chlorophyll molecule is markedly similar in its structure to the molecule in human blood called *heme* which hooks up with a protein to build the more familiar hemoglobin component of our blood. In the book *Cereal Grass, What's In It For You?* (Lawrence, KA: Wilderness Community Education Foundation, 1990, p.41), author Ronald Seibold writes:

> Perhaps the most interesting connection between green foods and blood is the similarity in the structures of the two colored pigments, heme and chlorophyll. The biological relationship between these two molecules, though studied for over 60 years, is still not completely clear. It does appear, however, that small amounts of the digestive products of chlorophyll may stimulate the synthesis of either heme or globin or both in animals and humans.

Anything that helps synthesize the heme or globin parts of our blood helps to build blood strength. I translate Seibold's statement to mean that the absorption of even small amounts of chlorophyll can build the health of the blood. A person of average health wouldn't have to eat large amounts of greens to reap great benefit. At least one serving a day would be a fine start. My twenty-five years of experience with using chlorophyll-rich, dark green foods, leaves no doubt that these foods can and do build the hemoglobin and many other components of healthy blood. The words "may stimulate," used by Seibold, are deliberately cautious. They do not communicate the full impact of what I have observed. (If I don't know *how* something works, I can still know *that* it works, right?)

All over the world, along with concern for cancer and other so-called "incurable" diseases, people are worried about radiation pollution whether from X-rays, high voltage power lines, computer screens or from nuclear discharges. Seibold discusses the power of green vegetables to protect against radiation damages of all types and to prevent diseases such as cancer. In reporting on the 1962 radiation research of Dr. Doris Calloway, who gave lethal doses of X-rays to mice, Seibold writes: "Ninety-seven percent of the mice given no vegetable supplements died within 20 days ... The dark green leafy vegetables provided, by far, the most protection from radiation." (p. 80) He goes on to say that within the same 20 days, only 12% of the animals who were fed mustard greens died. This is the kind of protection found in chlorophyll components.

Mr. Seibold also mentions the outstanding work of Dr. Chiu Nan Lai, at the University of Texas Medical Center, which shows that, "The more chlorophyll in the vegetable, the greater the protection from the carcinogen." (p. 43) The extensive list of the remarkable activities of chlorophyll is well documented in both scientific literature as well as in folk medicine.

If you are starting to believe in green power but are still in the grip of "I-am-not-used-to-the-taste-of-green," you can always get yourself some of the excellent green-food supplements available at health food stores. Two of my personal favorites are green tabs of *Wheat Grass* and *Barley Grass* from the Pines International, Inc., and a product called *Green Radiance* from Allergy Research/Nutricology, Inc.

No Folly in Folacin

Although the chlorophyll content of spinach is certainly nothing to sneeze at, other dark green leafy vegetables could have qualified for this slot on my *10 Essential Foods* list if chlorophyll were the final determining factor. Some of the other hypothetical competitors actually have slightly more beta carotene (kale), or more usable calcium (beet greens) than spinach (although spinach is also a prizewinner in the beta carotene department). However, spinach is unique among all leafy greens, in fact unique amongst most foods, for its extraordinary content of folacin (also called folic acid). Parsley is a close runner-up, but how often do we sit down to eat a bowl of parsley? All the other green foods have some folacin but not nearly the amount found in spinach.

Folacin is part of the B-vitamin complex. It has been singled out in health news more often in the past couple of years because it is now proven to be important in preventing birth defects, especially when used as a food supplement. But this is only a fragment of its fame in maintaining or rebuilding health.

Folacin:
- Is important in the breakdown and utilization of proteins.
- Helps form hemoglobin necessary for healthy red blood cells.
- Is essential for the processes of growth and reproduction of all body cells.
- Helps balance appetite and production of hydrochloric acid and this in turn works for preventing intestinal parasites and food poisoning.
- Aids in the performance of the liver.
- Prevents certain types of birth defects such as cleft palate, brain damage, and slow development or poor learning ability in the child.
- Protects against many types of cancers, especially lung, cervical and pancreatic.

Regarding cervical cancer, Jean Carper (in *Food Your Miracle Medicine*) confirms what I have read about folic acid and cervical cancer in several other resources. She reports on a virus which often leads to cervical cancer, noting that 80% of all cases of cervical cancer occur in women infected with this virus. Folic acid (at least 400 mcg. [micrograms] a day as researched by Dr. Charles Butterworth Jr., M.D. of the University of Alabama at Birmingham), can stop this virus and prevent it leading to cervical cancer. (However, if cervical cancer is already present, folic acid supplementation does not help.)

The amount of folic acid suggested as a preventive for cervical cancer (400 mcg. per day) is the basic amount suggested for all the benefits listed above. One serving (1 cup) of fresh spinach will give you at least 100 mcg. of folacin. A spinach salad of the size served at my favorite restaurant is about 2 cups of spinach (yes, it is huge!) so that means a hearty 200 mcg. input of folacin. Broccoli also has healthy amounts of folacin (approximately 71 mcg. in 1 cup), and the whole grains and beans have substantial amounts too. In fact, beans win a prize in the folacin department. One-half cup of cooked pinto beans contains approximately 146 mcg. of folacin.

No known toxicity level exists for folacin although the FDA limits folacin (folic acid) supplement tablets to 400 mcg. per tablet. Dr. Michael Colgan, director of the Colgan Institute of Nutritional Science in San Diego (and author of *The New Nutrition, Medicine For The Millennium*) emphatically suggests, along with his colleagues, that we need more folic acid than the 400 mcg. a day presently being claimed by some as a good maintenance level. Colgan points out that, "our own government surveys show widespread folic acid deficiencies in America which are getting worse by the decade as our food becomes ever more processed and degraded." (p. 83.)

By emphasizing the *10 Essential Foods* and their broader groups (as suggested under the Alternatives within each chapter), we can intelligently increase our intake of some of these crucial nutrients, such as folacin, which most Americans are deficient in.

The little hitch in all this good news about the folacin content of spinach and other foods is that folacin is a delicate nutrient. Cooking dramatically lessens its potency as does the improper storage of the fresh foods that contain it. Most folacin gets dumped down the drain with the cooking water in which it dissolved. It is damaged somewhat by the heat itself, and lessens if the fresh food is exposed to room temperature for prolonged periods. The bottom line is to buy fresh spinach, store it in a cool dark place like a refrigerator, and eat it soon while it is still fresh. Otherwise you might be faced with a wilted pile of green smelly stuff; as happened to a friend of mine who bought spinach with good intentions but forgot she had it in the refrigerator. (Check out ideas for the best ways of preparing spinach in the Shopping Skills section below.)

TASOLE: "This pregnancy is a little tougher than the last one," Gwen reported one day as we sat in her kitchen. "I am much more tired and moody. I wake up tired and its downhill from there. I certainly don't have the energy to play with Pam as often as she would like. She's just three you know, and she has bigger ideas than I can handle."

"What's your diet been like?" I asked.

"The usual. My diet is good actually—lots of fruits and vegetables; and my protein intake is up because the doctor suggested that might boost my energy."

"It doesn't sound like you are satisfied with the results yet," I replied, non-committally. "Is that all the doctor said?"

"He did a blood test and said I was very low in iron. He prescribed an iron supplement, but it doesn't seem to help and it definitely makes me constipated. I sure don't need that along with these pregnancy hemorrhoids. Thank God they only happen when I'm pregnant. Anyway, now I've stopped the iron supplements because they just add on another problem without helping the tiredness at all. While taking the iron supplements the doctor did another blood test after a week or so and it hadn't improved over the first test." Gwen did sound tired as she turned to me and asked, "Any ideas?"

Gwen was a woman who could make her own decisions when given basic information, so I told her what popped into my mind. "I learned a trick for this exact situation from a lay-midwife. I don't know if it would work for you, but it has worked in every case I've seen so far. How are you with green?"

"Green?" Gwen's left eyebrow went up so far it was hidden under her black bangs. (She can do that anytime she wants—I can't. My eyebrows seem determined to only work as a pair.)

"It's a drink," I explained. "I call it 'green drink' and I drink it all the time."

"I didn't know you were pregnant!" Gwen pretended in mock surprise. I have noticed over the years that we get in these odd moods together; getting less and less serious by the minute.

"You know I'm not pregnant," I chided. "Now listen up. This green drink is good for anybody at anytime, but I first learned about it from this midwife. I put into my blender about a cup of roughly-chopped fresh, raw spinach, preferably organic, along with maybe a fourth or half-cup of chopped parsley and then a small bunch of the fresh mint from my garden. I add a cup or so of pineapple juice—the exact amount depending on my mood; I don't actually measure any of these things. Then I blend it on the high-speed setting for about a minute, or until all the leaves are only tiny specks. What I end up with is a beautiful bright green mixture."

"Then what do you do with it?" Gwen asked hesitatingly.

"I drink it! It tastes wonderful—like pineapple-mint," I said enthusiastically until I saw the look on her face.

"I don't usually drink green liquids," Gwen stated firmly, wrinkling her nose. "I mean, how did you ever get around to liking to drink green stuff? This sounds to me like those blue pie crusts you told me you used to bake as a kid so the others wouldn't eat the pie and you could have it all for yourself."

The blue pie crust story was true and it made me smile that Gwen had remembered it. "It is quite easy to get used to this green drink because it tastes so great," I continued. "Let's go over to my house and make some and you can try it. I like lots of spinach and parsley in mine, but some people like a less concentrated green drink so I'll make a mild one for you, for starters. Everybody in my neighborhood enjoys green drinks now—babies, kids, in-laws, everyone! At first, some people said the same things as you, but they couldn't resist tasting it. After one taste you begin to get hooked."

On the way to my house Gwen asked, "What does this have to do with being tired and low-iron blood tests and the rest?"

I was reminded that I hadn't finished my story. "Oh, I forgot to tell you the rest of the midwife story. The point is that after even a *few* days of using green drink (maybe one or two cups a day although some loved it and drank more), every single woman had a significantly higher iron count without taking any supplements. Their general health always improved and tiredness vanished. Green drinks have all that chlorophyll, plus high amounts of beta carotene, minerals, folacin and other nutrients which absorb and go to work so easily. It makes a difference quickly. I think your doctor will be in for a big surprise on your next blood test if you'll try this idea."

By now we were at my house and I was whipping up a green drink. I often get carried away and end up with more in the blender that I can comfortably finish. "That's a lot of green drink," Gwen remarked, a bit nervously. "I'm not *that* thirsty," she continued hesitantly.

"Just take a taste and see what you think. I'll drink a bunch and have the rest at dinner if we have extra."

Just then the phone rang so I took my green drink into the other room where the telephone was, leaving Gwen in the kitchen with a tiny taste of green drink in her glass. I was on the telephone about ten minutes, which was longer than I had expected and long enough for me to have finished my drink. I strolled back into the kitchen to find another friend, Jim, finishing off the green drink with Gwen. She was smiling.

"It's definitely a winner!" Gwen announced confidently. "I was getting up my nerve to try it when Jim came in, saw the green drink and went for it right away. Being the competitive sort I grabbed it first, poured a small glass and started drinking. Was I ever pleasantly surprised!"

"Right!" Jim and Gwen were laughing together.

"Try drinking at least a cup or two every day until your next blood test and see what happens." I looked at Gwen.

"I don't see what this could hurt," Gwen responded. "I really do like it. Can a person drink too much of it?"

"Probably so. Chlorophyll cleanses the blood of toxins and can be quite stimulating to the entire system. Some people should go slower with that kind of cleansing action. I do know at least one person who has overdone it on occasion," I looked knowingly at Jim. "That person began drinking a quart a day before he had gotten used to it, and that's a lot even for die-hards like me. Anyway, the person will remain anonymous but suffice it to say there was a marked increase in trips to the toilet. I believe it's called *diarrhea*."

About ten days later Gwen called to report on her doctor visit. "My blood test was so different he insisted on doing it twice. Then he remarked on how he had never seen those iron tablets work that well before." Gwen chuckled. "When I told him I hadn't taken any for more than two weeks I think he was torn between annoyance and curiosity. When I told him about green drinks he didn't seem interested in the details but just said to keep on with whatever I was doing because it was helping significantly. Of course, that's what I plan to do. My family is starting to get hooked too. It's unbelievable."

"What about the tiredness and low moods?" I questioned.

"All gone after two days of green drinks. I'm even starting to make mine greener, like you do. My hemorrhoids are definitely improving except on the uh ...well the uh ... the day that I overdid the green drink like that other friend you mentioned. I guess diarrhea isn't the most helpful for hemorrhoids, but that was only once and now I just stick to one or two cups a day. [*How's that for a misplaced modifier?* — Editor] Even my eyes seem less strained from all the reading I do. Could the green drinks be helping all that?"

"Sure. That's why I drink it. Not everyday at the moment, but once or twice a week. Green drink is a tasty way to have a tonic." Talking about green drinks made me want some. So as I finished our talk I headed straight for the mint patch and then for the kitchen.

As I told Gwen, it is possible to overdo it on green foods when you use them in such a concentrated form as a green drink. However, it is fairly impossible to overdo it simply by eating greens as part of a daily meal.

Trouble With Oxalic?

Some critics argue that spinach has a drawback in its structure because of a component called oxalic acid. While it is true that oxalic acid combines with some of the iron and calcium in the spinach, limiting the amount of these minerals the body can absorb, oxalic acid does not block all mineral absorption. Since spinach has so many other outstanding properties (i.e. the ability of its chlorophyll to build the heme and globin parts of blood), I don't consider this "oxalic acid thing" a problem at all. For extra calcium and iron, go for the Figs, Carrots, grains and all the rest of the *10 Essential Foods*, and keep spinach on the pedestal it deserves. (By the way, as I mentioned in the Dulse chapter, for those of you following the pop medical advice to eat certain chewable antacid tablets as a cheap calcium source, be warned that oxalic acid pales in comparison to these products in making calcium unavailable. I repeat, unavailable! These antacid products have lots of calcium, yes. But this type of calcium neutralizes your stomach acid, which is the job it is made for; and without stomach acid working, no calcium can be broken down and absorbed—nor can many other nutrients! In my observation this type of calcium will simply "gum up" your digestive tract and your overall health, in the long run. As calcium supplements, certain antacids are worse than no calcium at all!)

While I am on this subject of the oxalic acid in spinach I will tell you a bit of esoterica I learned from one of my main teachers of the healing arts—and believe me she really knew what she was doing! That woman had twelve wonderful children and could heal everything from scraped knees to gangrene with herbs and all sorts of other self-help means. She and her husband were two of the most talented healers I have ever met, and I have met many. In addition to alternative healing skills, she taught me (and hundreds of others) about the healing and rejuvenating properties of food. Although she did not bother much with offering scientific proof for her "food healing" information, when she told me that the oxalic acid in raw spinach had powerful healing properties (particularly for tumors) when not cooked, I took it to heart and still do to this day. She said the same thing about the oxalic acid in raw asparagus too, and never let her apprentices eat either vegetable in a cooked form. So, I say "Who cares ..." if oxalic acid in spinach blocks some of the absorption of iron and calcium. The other advantages far outweigh this problem.

Potassium Rich

Don't worry about the oxalic acid blocking all the rest of the minerals and other remarkably good stuff in spinach. It does not. Spinach is considered a "potassium food," for instance, and is one of the foods that can contribute significantly to the daily potassium intake (an extra daily intake of 400 mg. potassium, or 3/4 cup cooked fresh spinach) known to slash the odds of having a fatal stroke by 40%. Potassium is also crucial for transmitting nerve impulses, regulating body fluids, normalizing heartbeat, nourishing the muscles ... and so many other things. (I'm just mentioning a few teasers.) So go ahead— knock yourself out and eat your potassium foods every day. (These include *all vegetables* by the way, especially the dark green leafy vegetables; and Figs are great too.).

Better Beta

Spinach is outstanding in beta carotene content. I wrote more thoroughly about the lifegiving properties of beta carotene in the Carrot chapter, so I will only make a short accounting here. Beta carotene is a highly active antioxidant showing properties that: prevent cancer tissue from growing, build the immune system, slash the potential for having a stroke, protect the health of arteries, and fight infection. Spinach and Carrots are so high in this component that they were actually named specifically in a Harvard study as two foods with enough beta carotene to diminish the possibility of stroke by 40%. The dietary suggestion from the study was to eat three cups of spinach, cooked or raw, or one and a half carrots a day. (study quoted in *Food Your Miracle Medicine*, p. 98. See Recommended Bibliography.)

More About Phytos

Lutein and zeaxanthin are two more of the antioxidant phytochemicals present in highest amounts in dark green leafy vegetables including spinach. In fact, lutein is showing itself to be as amazing as beta carotene and already it is being marketed as a food supplement from the carotenoid group. As I reiterate throughout this book, these antioxidants/phytochemicals, which are abundant in fresh foods, catalyze, preserve, and rejuvenate health more powerfully than many so called "miracle drugs." No diet is "top notch" without them, and the more foods are processed, the less phytochemicals they have.

In the May 15, 1995 issue of *U.S. News & World Report*, there is a full color, two page spread titled "New Powers of Produce: Looking beyond beta carotene," about the healing potential of phytochemicals. Several of my *10 Essential Foods* were mentioned specifically as outstanding choices. About spinach, the author Susan Brink says: "Spinach...is loaded with lutein and zeaxanthin which cut the risk of blindness due to age-related macular degeneration—possibly by protecting the blood vessels that supply the retinas. Researchers recommend at least one weekly serving." (Lalitha recommends more than that of course!).

The magazine *Dynamic Chiropractic* (April 24, 1995) listed a phytochemical review which showed that lutein and zeaxanthin reduce the incidence of cataracts.

Keeping in mind that all the functional components of a fresh food work synergistically with one another and so are at peak efficiency when ingested in whole food form, we should hold ourselves back as much as possible from the urge to simply use supplements.

SHOPPING FOR SPINACH and OTHER FOOD SKILLS

Color is the first thing to look for when shopping for great spinach. No yellow tinges for you! Get the darkest green bunch and don't accept any hint of wilt. Always buy organic spinach if you can because if it's not organic it has a high probability of being sprayed with several (if not all) of the ten different, significantly nasty, agricultural poisons/contaminants reported by David Steinman and Samuel Epstein, authors of the highly trustworthy and meticulously researched book, *The Safe Shopper's Bible* (New York, NY: Macmillan, 1995). If you can't get organic spinach, remember to use the detox method I describe in chapter 2. The detox-soak, along with the wash, can help reduce pesticides/contaminants from the surface of the leaves. (Don't get totally discouraged with all this contamination talk. Remember, the functional components in spinach, even when it is not organic, are so powerful in promoting health and well-being that the bottom line in any case is to "eat green.")

It is so easy to grow green foods such as spinach, (and Sprouts) that even if you live in a city, and even if it is the middle of winter, you can decorate your windowsills with pots of growing spinach, or alfalfa or sunflower seed Sprouts, and snack away all year long.

Spinach often requires careful washing because of the tricky way it can hide bits of dirt from the farm. However, the best time to wash it is no more than a couple of days before you intend to use it; after washing the natural wilt and decay process is speeded up. (When I pick spinach off the plants in my garden it is usually so clean that I rarely need to wash it at all, which is ideal as there are delicate oils on fresh leaves that are wasted in the rinsing or washing process.)

To "quick cook" spinach for best retention of functional components use a vegetable steamer basket that elevates your vegetables above the water. Steam for just two minutes or so.

HEALTHY ADDITIONS, ALTERNATIVES and TRAVELERS TIPS

Top Alternatives to spinach are parsley, chard and kale. However, the Addition of any dark leafy greens to your diet is worth pursuing tenaciously.

For those of you who want additional green in your diet besides what you already eat, there are some ingeniously prepared green-food concentrates at your health food store. Yes,

I'm saying you can theoretically get many of the significant health benefits of live food by taking a supplement. Of course you miss all the enjoyment of munching a luscious spinach salad, for instance, but hey, it's still a worthwhile Alternative. People in ill health who need concentrated "green help" may especially profit from green foods supplements. Three of the best I have found are *Phyt-Aloe* (chewable or capsule) sold mail-order by the Rejenitec company, whole leaf *Wheat Grass* or *Barley Grass* produced by the Pines company, and *Green Radiance* from Nutricology Inc. (See more information about these foods under Healthy Additions in the Broccoli chapter; and also in Supplies Appendix B.)

For travelers, properly dehydrated greens could be a way to add more spinach or other greens into your diet in soups and other dishes, if you are in a position to cook for yourself. Sporting goods stores that cater to backpackers and health food stores carry dehydrated vegetables of varying variety. Remember that Dulse and other sea vegetables are great choices for traveling foods of the leafy variety. Growing Sprouts in a traveling "Sprout bag" has worked well for me on many a trip. It could work for you too. (See the TASOLE in the Sprouts chapter, about making Sprouts while in India.)

When traveling far from home and perhaps even far from modern grocery stores, go to the open air markets and choose the locally grown fresh greens. In some countries, such as India, fresh foods should usually, unfortunately, be cooked or peeled to help eliminate some of the airborne contaminants such as parasites. When I travel, I always take Grapefruit extract so that I can detox my fresh foods when I need to.

SURVIVAL CHOICES for COMPROMISING CIRCUMSTANCES

You may have to go for the frozen spinach which (unlike canned spinach) at least has an adequate amount of nutrients preserved. However, canned spinach is better than eating no spinach at all.

In a restaurant, order a spinach salad or Caesar salad, as the fresh greens involved in these salads are far better nutritionally than the wimpy iceberg lettuce salads usually offered.

Cooked spinach in a restaurant dish, such as the delicious *sag paneer* found in Indian restaurants, or spinach lasagna or quiche, are possible restaurant choices that can still reap some benefits for you from the minerals and fiber. (But they won't replace the additional fresh greens you are ordering—right?) Steamed fresh greens such as spinach, chard or kale are excellent restaurant choices.

For those using frozen dinners, buy those that contain green foods such as spinach, kale, chard, green beans and Broccoli. Organic-food frozen dinners are available at some health stores. These are of varying quality, can offer some nutrition, but would still be a low priority. Just do the best you can.

Dehydrated greens are a good choice as I mentioned in the Healthy Additions. I've put them in this section also because they can store for long periods, thus becoming a healthy choice for a "survival food." Such greens may go a long way to preserving your health in an emergency situation.

During a busy work day or when traveling, it is worth considering investing in a green supplement, such as one of the two types I have suggested earlier.

KIDS LOVE THIS

Children enjoy the "green drinks" I describe in the TASOLE above, especially if there is no authority figure around passing on a "green phobia." For children, or anyone new to this food item, make the drink with more pineapple juice and less greens, perhaps only three or four spinach leaves to start with and a sprig of fresh mint. Babies often love diluted green drink in their bottles, but you have to strain it first or the plant fibers block the bottle nipple! Frozen green drinks make tasty popsicle treats, especially in the summer.

Another green recipe:

RAW SPINACH SOUP (makes 3 cups)

Blend well in the blender:
1/4 cup almonds
1 cup tomato juice
1 cup water
2 cups raw spinach
1 small clove garlic, minced
1 Tbs. chopped scallion (1 thin scallion)
1/2 cup packed celery leaves
3/8 tsp. ground cumin (or) 1/8 tsp. ground nutmeg
1/8 tsp. kelp or dulse powder, or vegetable salt

After blending the above mixture, gradually add and blend in a second cup of water, blending to the consistency you like.

Note that the taste will be completely different if you use nutmeg in place of cumin. If you aren't sure which to use, empty small amounts of the mixture into two cups. Then add a pinch of nutmeg to one cup and two pinches of cumin to the other. They are both good!

Recipes from: Nostrand, Carol. *Junk Food to Real Food* (New Caanan, CT: Keats Publishing 1994, p. 170). Used with permission.

ALFALFA CROQUETTES (serves 2)

Mix thoroughly:
1 cup alfalfa sprouts
2 Tbs. grated red cabbage
2 Tbs. grated carrot
4 Tbs. chopped celery
2 Tbs. chopped parsley
1/2 tsp. minced garlic
2 Tbs. tahini [sesame seed spread]
3 Tbs. carrot juice
1 tsp. lemon juice
1/2 cup ground sunflower seeds
(about 1/3 cup unground seeds)

Serving Suggestions:
Serve in tomato cups. Cut the tomato about 3/4 of the way down, 3 ways, so that you have 6 sections connected at the bottom. After you fill them with the mixture, top with parsley sprigs and serve on a bed of lettuce.

(or)

Refrigerate the mixture for 1 hour, so that it is more stiff, then form patties.

Recipe from: Nostrand, Carol. *Junk Food to Real Food* (New Caanan, CT: Keats Publishing, 1994, p. 180). Used with permission.

FUNCTIONAL COMPONENTS
in 100 Grams Alfalfa Sprouts
Serving Size: 1 cup, 33 grams, raw alfalfa sprouts

Calories	29.0
Protein	4.g
Fat	.69g
Carbohydrates	3.78g
Fiber	1.64g
Cholesterol	0
Calcium	32.0 mg
Phosphorus	70.0 mg
Magnesium	27.0 mg
Potassium	79.0 mg
Sodium	6.0 mg
Iron	.96 mg
Copper	.157 mg
Manganese	.188 mg
Zinc	.92 mg
Selenium	n/a
Chromium	n/a
Vitamin A	155. mg
Vitamin C	8.2 mg
Vitamin B1 (Thiamin)	.076 mg
Vitamin B2 (Riboflavin)	.126 mg
Vitamin B3 (Niacin)	.481 mg
Vitamin B6	.034 mg
Folacin	36.0 mcg
Vitamin B12	0
Pantothenic Acid (Vit. B5)	.563
Vitamin E	trace
Biotin	trace

Prominent Phytochemicals and Antioxidants in Sprouts:
Beta carotene, vitamin C, trace minerals, chlorophyll, plus antioxidants specific to each type of sprouted plant.

Sources:
1) Santillo, Humbart, N.D. *Intuitive Eating* (Prescott, AZ: Hohm Press, 1993).
2) Balch, Phyllis A., C.N.C. and James F., M.D. *Prescription for Cooking* (Greenfield, IN: PAB Books, 1987.)
3) Margen, Sheldon, M.D. and the Editors of the University of California at Berkeley "Wellness Newsletter," *The Wellness Encyclopedia of Food and Nutrition* (New York, NY: Rebus Press [Random House], 1992).

12

SPROUTS

WHAT IS SO GOOD ABOUT SPROUTS?

Sprouts are the brand new little babies of food plants. Just think of it! Homegrown and store-bought sprouts, popping out of the seed, are full of the life force of creation—unspoiled, unsprayed with pesticides or herbicides, unfertilized, unpreserved, and naturally organic because all you do to them is rinse with pure water and make sure they drain properly. Their life-embracing systems are turned up for peak performance. As these vibrant sprouting tots race their way to adulthood, Nip! Here comes the sprout lover to eat this super-concentrated vitality as a sort of rocket-fuel food for health!

Alfalfa sprouts are my sprout-of-choice amongst many wonderful sprout possibilities. This is because alfalfa sprouts are widely liked and probably the most familiar. Alfalfa seeds are also affordable and easily available, and any "klutz" can grow them in a tiny space (a small bamboo basket would be ideal) with hardly any fuss at all. Alfalfa sprouts are generally available ready-to-eat, even in ordinary grocery stores, and will probably be the sprout that most people will try first. However, for the purposes of *10 Essential Foods* I include the *whole category of sprouts* and will therefore be mentioning lots of others in addition to my main example of alfalfa sprouts.

Nutrient content is an outstanding trait of sprouts, despite what "sprout criticizers" say regarding sprouts being too small and undeveloped to provide much. This is definitely an uninformed rumor. Seeds hold a magnificent concentration of vitamins, minerals, proteins, enzymes, and fatty acids which begin multiplying "like crazy" when a seed germinates. Germination is the magical moment when a seed goes from "hibernation" into the active process of sprouting and then growing into a mature plant. Very often all it takes is the addition of water to a seed to initiate the germination process. In his book *Sprouts the Miracle Food* (Great Barrington, MA: The Sprout House Inc., 1997, p. 93), author and American folk hero for sprouts, Steve Meyerowitz (known world-wide as "Sproutman"), lists some of the miracles that are initiated with germination:

- Nutrients are broken down and simplified [through enzymatic action]: protein into amino acids, fats into essential fatty acids, starches to sugars and minerals chelate or combine with protein in a way that increases their utilization. These processes all increase nutrition and improve digestion and assimilation. This is the reason sprouts are considered predigested food.
- Proteins, vitamins, enzymes, minerals, and trace minerals multiply from 300 to 1200 percent.
- Chlorophyll develops in green plants.
- Certain acids and toxins which ordinarily would interfere with digestion are reduced and/or eliminated
- Size and water content increase dramatically.

"Sproutman" healed himself of lifelong allergies and asthma through restructuring his diet and adding lots of these lively sprouts. He writes:

> Since I lived in an apartment, I learned to garden indoors. Before long I was dining on crisp *Chinese cabbage, luscious crimson clover, hearty sunflower, succulent buckwheat lettuce, spicy red radish, velvety kale, sweet green pea*—I had so much, I fed all my friends and students. These young greens were so alive and scintillating with color and aroma, you could practically feel their vitamins! Make no mistake about it. That

vitality is assimilated by *you*—in the form of active enzymes, vitamins, amino acids, trace minerals, RNA, DNA, oxygen and other secret elements about which only nature knows. You can't buy that nutrition in a pill! (p. 2)

One outstanding trait of sprouts has become the subject of some controversy. As sprouts have highly-energetic enzyme activity, the controversy centers around whether or not these food enzymes can enhance digestive processes in those who eat them. The same controversy, by the way, applies to all raw foods in general, although sprouts are exceptionally hot in enzyme activity (as growing things are known to be). The arguments of a couple of food experts will illustrate this point.

In his book, *Food Enzymes The Missing Link To Radiant Health* (Prescott, AZ: Hohm Press, 1987, p. 31), Humbart Santillo, N.D., in speaking of raw foods, says, "It is a fact that the enzymes in foods aid in digestion." Santillo's entire book is a very convincing compilation of scientific evidence to support this, and his work as a health professional also bears this out.

Ron Seibold, in *Cereal Grass: What's In It For You?* (Lawrence, KA: Wilderness Community Education Foundation, 1990, pp. 76-77), highly praises the benefits of raw foods and the great vitality to be found in green cereal grass juices which are like a "virtual enzyme factory." However, although he does say that taking a digestive enzyme supplement could be helpful to some people, he also clearly states that "... enzymes in foods have little to do with enzymes needed in our bodies," and " ... few of the enzymes available in whole foods function as digestive enzymes." Seibold's arguments also sound well-considered and substantiated.

Because of my own overwhelmingly positive experiences with the digestive enhancement and nutritional availability afforded through the eating of raw foods, sprouts, and raw juices, I have to agree with Dr. Santillo's stand on the case. I also have to say, however, that I won't be surprised to find out that both are right and that the so-called controversy is only a lack of information. (In situations like this, I often start off knowing *that* something is, but maybe not exactly *how* or *why* the thing is.)

For those of you who enjoy anecdotal evidence, I can report that one of my primary teachers in the healing arts, who was incredibly psychic, told me she could *see* the enzymes from live food actually going to work in people. She said it looked to her as though highly beneficial, yet subtle, life energies were "guided" or directed by the physical enzymes. For those who ate the live foods, this partnership of energy and enzymes enlivened far more benefits than just the physical digestive help of the food enzymes. She always insisted that her apprentices eat lots of sprouts in great variety. In fact, one of my responsibilities was to grow sprouts for our whole group.

So, from the premise that the enzymes in sprouts (and to varying degrees in other raw plants) can indeed help our health, I will explain a little of how this probably comes about, at least on the physical level. (Of course I'll be explaining "Lalitha style." While I like my own style and know it to be accurate for its purpose, some of you may want to get a more comprehensive approach by reading the two books mentioned above, or some of the source matter they refer to.)

How Sprouts Work

In both people and plants, all types of enzymes work directly or indirectly to turn nutrients into catalytic substances for sustaining all "bodily" functions and thus creating vibrant health. In people, some enzymes such as *digestive enzymes* break down various components of the foods we eat. These components, in turn, are necessary to *metabolic enzymes* in doing their jobs (although all enzyme jobs are happening simultaneously of course).

A deficiency in enzymes equals a deficiency in health. Even though we do have a reserve supply of enzymes which we are born with, and, in addition, some of our organs are responsible for making specific enzymes (for instance the healthy pancreas makes enzymes for use in the stomach), we can also add to our digestive enzyme activity through the raw foods we eat, or by ingesting enzyme supplements made from raw foods. Eating sprouts, for instance, greatly enhances our digestive potential with their own enzymes, enabling us to use less of our valuable reserves. The more enzymes we add to the digestive process from the outside (via raw foods) the less our bodies have to spend their energies making digestive enzymes of their own. In *Intuitive Eating* (p. 284) (see Recommended Bibliography), Dr. Humbart Santillo explains it this way:

> Food sits in our cardiac (upper part of our stomach), or pre-digestive stomach, for 30-60 minutes before enzymes are secreted to it. If the food

is raw, the enzymes already contained in the food can actually digest a percentage of the food within this part of the stomach. This takes the stress off the pancreas. The pancreas will not have to produce and secrete as many enzymes to digest the whole food because it is partially digested. This saves the pancreas from enzyme exhaustion and strengthens the immune system.

Additionally, many people are so weak in their ability to produce digestive enzymes in the first place, that this raw-food enzyme help can make a huge difference in nutrient availability for all other body processes. Further, this conservation of resources not only leaves the body with more energy available for producing the thousands of other types of enzymes it needs, but also enhances the availability of the myriad nutrients which are crucial to that "enzyme factory" with which the body sustains its life.

Without the entire enzyme process working efficiently, lots of tiresome and aggravating health problems are further exaggerated and perhaps prevented from healing. A few of the illnesses which are aggravated or perhaps caused through enzyme insufficiency include allergies of all sorts, skin problems, low immunity, and kidney weakness (caused by toxic overload in the blood causing the kidneys to have to work too hard).

Not only do raw foods and fresh raw juices contribute to the digestive enzyme supply that the body is also producing, with sprouts there is another highly desirable enzyme activity happening. As sprouts begin to grow, their enzymes are highly activated to *predigest* many of the nutrients in their seeds. For instance, starches, proteins and fats are broken down into simpler components within the sprouting seed so that the sprout can convert them into different components needed for further growth. In this growth-oriented process, which slows down as plants mature, sprouts are a powerhouse of predigested nutrients that become readily available to us when we eat the sprouts.

Many factors—such as a diet high in cooked and processed foods (heat and/or processing "kills" enzyme activity), emotional upset, fatigue, environmental pollution, contaminated food, stressful work conditions, or even a high-intensity physical work-out—contribute to depleting all types of our enzyme supplies. Symptoms of aging, like the wearing out of the body, are synonymous with that depletion. When we eat raw foods we directly replenish the digestive part of the enzyme pool while enhancing the action of other enzyme types indirectly through nutrient availability.

The unhappy news is that many of us have such a deficit of digestive enzyme activity that no matter *what* we eat it simply gallops down the esophagus to land "unattended" in the stomach, where a literal "toxic rotting process" begins. Bad breath, gas, fatigue, indigestion symptoms of all sorts and even bad moods are a few of the possible indicators of such poor digestion. The poisons from this undigested or incompletely digested food have to be dealt with by the liver, kidneys, and other processes of detoxification that themselves need enzymes to work properly. In a depleted system the poisons are simply kept recycling in a survival holding-pattern that can only contribute to the further deterioration of health and the headlong rush into the breakdown that some people wrongly assume is "natural" old age.

Many healing therapies are firmly based in rejuvenating health and even slowing (what I call "harmonizing") the processes of aging through the use of raw foods, sprouts, and fresh raw juices. In addition to the seemingly limitless array of healing phytochemicals and other functional components which I keep talking about throughout this book, the enzyme availability in those foods significantly adds to this rejuvenation and harmonization. I continually suggest we eat *live* foods, especially sprouts, every day, and thus prevent the horror story which I described above.

TWO TYPES

There are two basic types of sprouts: 1. The type that are sprouted in about 5-10 days: the grower intends them to form a delicate, tender, chlorophyll-rich green leaf structure such as alfalfa, radish and sunflower sprouts. Therefore these are usually grown upright for best results. And 2. The type that are sprouted in about 3 to 6 days—the grower does not intend these to form a green leaf structure but rather a short sprouted "tail" perhaps up to 1/2 inch long. These second types are usually sprouted beans or grains such as wheat, lentils, flax, or pinto beans and are often grown in a jar, plastic container, or a natural-fiber cloth bag. (I use flax-cloth.)

Most seeds are traditionally grown one way or the other for best results. However there are some, such as buckwheat,

Sprouts: The Most Nutritious Vegetables on the Planet

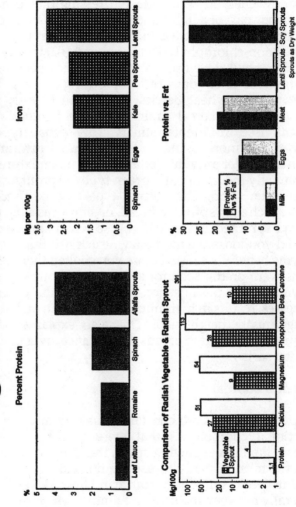

figure 12.1 Charts Compiled by Steve Meyerowitz, author of *Sprouts The Miracle Food*, using USDA data

which can be grown as a short-tail sprouted grain, or as a green leaf sprout. For those who wish to become accomplished sprout-growers, these finer points of spouting are explained in *Sprouts the Miracle Food!* (see Recommended Bibliography).

The "chlorophyll type" of sprouts (#1) need sunlight to mature properly, and are meant to be eaten raw in salads and on sandwiches, etc. With a tasty dressing they can even make up a major part of a light lunch. (You may wish to read over the chlorophyll research cited in the Spinach chapter.)

The "non-chlorophyll type" of sprout (#2) is not sprouted for its chlorophyll development and does not need any sunlight for the three to six days of its sprouting process. This second type includes wheat berries, lentils, chick peas, green peas, many types of cereal grains and the familiar mung bean sprouts used in Oriental stir-fry. This second type are much heavier and more filling and, when eaten raw, are generally eaten in smaller amounts, often as part of a mixture that is predominantly the lighter and green type of sprout, or as part of a leafy green salad. This second type may be used in cooked forms, such as in sprouted bread, or simply as a big pot of slow-cooked sprouted beans. (Of course when sprouted beans are cooked you loose the food enzyme activity, but you still get an enzyme benefit because, before you cooked them, the sprouted beans were predigested for at least a day or two by their own enzymes. This predigestion, along with the other sprouting processes, results in their nutritional content, including protein, being greatly heightened. This also explains why I prefer sprouted whole-grain breads, for instance, over their flour-only counterparts.)

Protein Potential

Sprouting seeds are constantly making more protein out of functional components that were stored within the seed. During the initial growing spurt, this protein content, some of it in the form of ready-to-use amino acids, keeps multiplying until it "peaks out" (as Sproutman Steve Meyerowitz puts it), generally between the fifth and ninth days. Sprouts are regular protein factories, pumping out this highly-prized nutrient in a user-friendly form. Not only that, but the sprout is also pumping out the vitamins and minerals necessary for the building and assimilation of the protein, developing chlorophyll (if it is the green-leaf type sprout) and producing high-quality predigested carbohydrates too. This predigested carbohydrate production is especially true with the bean and grain sprouts! I'm telling you—this business of eating the babies of plants just might be the tapping of the proverbial Fountain of Youth! Wahoo! Yipee! And to think you can grow them abundantly and inexpensively anywhere in the world, in one square foot of space or less!

TASOLE: I have become quite expert at growing sprouts for myself, both at home and whenever I travel. Even if I'm in a place where the water might be contaminated, and therefore suspicious for use in sprout growing, I have my "little ways" of making good out of the situation.

Once, traveling in India, I was feeling a little nutritionally deprived after a couple months of back-country fare in smaller villages. Right about that time, however, it became necessary for me to go into Pondicherry, a city on the southeastern coast. With fantasies of sprouts filling my imagination, I headed straight for one of the fabulous open-air food markets where I hoped to find suitable seeds. Near the edge of the flower market, where I nearly got permanently intoxicated by the delicious fragrance of the fresh flowers, I stumbled into the stall of a dried-bean salesman and found what I was looking for. Lentils! What luck!

Buying a small newspaper-wrapped packet of lentil seeds (the green kind many of us make lentil soup out of) I hurried off to find a room at one of the many inexpensive hostels near the ocean. On my way I bought a bottle of purified water for use in getting my sprouts started without delay. In my backpack I found a thin disposable plastic cup from a hostel I had stayed at some months back, battered but not leaking yet (the cup that is). I also pulled out of the depths of my pack one fairly new (surprise!) zip-lock baggie which I had brought from home. With these necessities I was ready. I filled the plastic cup one-third full with lentils and two-thirds with water, and left the mixture to soak while I took off for the boardwalk along the ocean to see the sights.

The next morning I poured off the water that the lentils had soaked overnight in (I always poured it on a needy potted plant of which there were many at this hostel), rinsed the soaked lentils in as small an amount of fresh bottled water as necessary, then left the now plump lentils in their cup to start sprouting as I took off for the day's adventures.

In order to get out of the area of my hostel, it was most interesting to go each day through a large temple which was always surrounded by the same band of well-fed beggars. Different members of the band had their own corners to attend to, and my favorite group was comprised of five very old women all of whom had few, if any, teeth. These women grinned magnanimously from their places in the gutter each time they saw me pass by. If I happened to be eating anything as I walked through, they of course would hold out their hands to beg for some of it, and I could never refuse their requests. Their enthusiasm for my approach increased each day since I never showed up empty-handed. It was a fine arrangement all around.

One woman in particular became more intimate with me through glance, silent gesture or nod as my twice-a-day passings proceeded. She seemed to be in charge of the others, seemed older by far, and was always allowed (expected?) by the others to take the food from me and eat first, before passing it to the other eager hands of her cadre.

Meanwhile, each day I would never neglect to rinse, at least once and sometimes twice, my prized lentil sprouts which were popping open (sprouting) beautifully in their plastic cup on my bedroom table top. The lentils were sprouting so well, in fact, that on day two, after the initial overnight soaking, I transferred the sprouting lentils into the plastic baggie (which I left open so the sprouts could "breathe") to continue sprouting, while I started another small batch soaking in the plastic cup. In this way, by day three after the initial soaking, I had a good two handfuls of perfectly sprouted lentils—my idea of a fantastic power-snack, full of the nutrients I had been craving. That morning, I savored my lentil sprout snack—sprout by carefully tended sprout—as I prepared for the day's wanderings and was still popping them bit by bit into my mouth as I approached the temple. About a block away from the temple I put the remaining lentils into a small pouch I always carried and made ready for the old women beggars with some bread rolls I had purchased on the way (I knew the women could easily eat and would like these.)

The head woman happily took the rolls and passed them out to the eagerly reaching hands of the others. Then she turned back to me and shyly tapped on the small pouch that hung at my side. Apparently she had seen me putting sprouts into my mouth as I had approached and had also observed me putting that "mysterious something" into the pouch before offering her the bread. Now she wanted to eat what I had been eating and she knew it was in the pouch.

From my experience I was fairly certain that she was not going to like the sprouts and I didn't want them to be fed to the cows. (Cows were waiting nearby, as they almost always are on the streets of India.) I brought out the sprouts and put one into her hand while trying to tell her with gesture and facial expression how crisp it was and the fact that it would be hard for her to chew properly. (She had few teeth, remember.) The old beggar stared curiously at the sprout in her hand and gestured that she wanted another, so I handed her a few more. She held the sprouts possessively but didn't eat them as she shook her head, staring more closely first at the sprouts and then at me. Finally, she placed them back in my palm and I started to walk away, throwing those few well-handled sprouts to the waiting cows.

Several yards down the street, I reached into my pouch for another sprout munch as I walked along. Within seconds, the entire group of beggar ladies had popped up from their temple-side seats and rushed towards me with their hands out. They had been watching me closely and when they saw my hand go from pouch to mouth they were now sure they had missed out on something. Politely but firmly they insisted on seeing the sprouts once again, so I produced a few more and put them into the head lady's hand as I had done before. Eyeing me intently she gestured for me to eat one so she could see how it was done. I took a few sprouts from my pouch, popped them into my mouth, and proceeded chewing with my usual pleasure. The head lady followed my lead, chewing as best she could. With a big smile on her face she turned to show off to the others. As the moments passed, with she and I chewing our sprouts, her smile quickly faded. Next, a look of chagrin, and then one of complete disapproval as she spat the remains of the sprouts into the street, where they were quickly lapped up by a passing cow.

I'll never forget the look those beggar women gave me as they marched indignantly back to their seats by the temple sidewalk. My highly-prized lentil sprouts found no appreciation from them. How does the old saying go? Is it "One woman's trash is another woman's treasure?"

Isn't that just the way!

SPROUT WARNING! FACT OR FICTION?

In case you may have heard bad press along the lines of: "Don't eat sprouts because many types are poisonous," I would like to address that issue here. One such incident involved the phytochemical L-canavanine in alfalfa seed. Stated briefly, the story goes that in the early 1980s scientists, including Dr. Emil J. Bardana working with Dr. René Malinow, wanted to show that high concentrations of L-canavanine could be connected to the development of lupus. This was proven, and the headlines hit the news that eating sprouts could be a hazard to health. What these headlines didn't say was that the so-called incriminating data on alfalfa (which spilled over, by misinformed inference, onto other sprouts) resulted from the ingestion of large amounts of dehydrated, barely germinated *seeds*. This is not the form that is ever typically consumed by humans. (I ask you, who in their right mind is going to eat large amounts of nasty-tasting, dried and ground up, barely-germinated alfalfa seed? In order to get the test-monkeys to eat it I bet the researchers had to trick them.)

Steve Meyerowitz, author of *Sprouts the Miracle Food!*, who talked about this issue to Dr. Bardana personally, noted that the "... monkeys, rodents and rabbits were fed biscuits made from alfalfa seed as well as alfalfa meal from alfalfa hay and tablets containing high doses of L-Canavanine sulfate" (p.115); whereas alfalfa seeds grown for typical sprout consumption would be sprouted for an average of seven days and by that time, Meyerowitz explained, there would be no L-canavanine left as a result of the sprouting process itself!

LALITHA RANTS: The point is that mature alfalfa sprouts are a wonderful and super-charged food. Barely germinated seeds, dried and concentrated into an unpalatable meal are NOT! A news story about sprouts that can be turned into a sensational scare, however temporary, is probably quite profitable for those who print it. If we did not have brains to think for ourselves, by now we would have eliminated tomatoes, mushrooms, several types of beans, and even black pepper from our diets because of similar renditions of so-called scientific research on plant toxins!

A final word on this unfortunate "sprout-rumor-gone-wild" is that Dr. Bardana himself told Steve Meyerowitz that there was no basis to the claim that eating alfalfa sprouts would cause lupus. "I wouldn't discourage my lupus patients from eating alfalfa sprouts," Bardana concluded. Well whatdya-know!

SHOPPING FOR SPROUTS and OTHER FOOD SKILLS

I'm not claiming that we have to eat bushels of sprouts every day. Some days eat a whole sprout salad, some days eat sprouts as part of a sandwich, some days eat them as sprouted whole grain bread. (Yes, there is such a yummy thing. One type tastes like a thick, sticky, sweet cake. My favorite brand of that particular type is Nature's Path *Manna Bread*, rye carrot raisin flavor. For a sprouted grain bread that is more like the ordinary sliced bread we are used to, I like *Ezekiel Bread*, made by Food For Life.) Some days you may eat no sprouts at all but you might be including other raw foods or fresh juice, just to let your body know you are still interested in contributing. Right?

If you are new at eating sprouts, I highly suggest starting off with alfalfa, sunflower, and/or radish sprouts whether you are growing your own or buying them at the store. These three types are most often eaten raw in salads, on sandwiches, as garnishes, or in place of fresh greens.

You are also likely to see various larger-type bean sprouts for sale such as lentils, garbonzos (chick peas), peas, red beans, kidney beans and mungs. These heavier sprouts can be eaten raw, often in smaller quantities and less frequently than the lighter green-leaf types, or cooked in various dishes.

Consumers can buy seeds for sprouting which are specially quality-controlled and mechanically sorted. This means that you will get a higher percentage of germination and less "clinkers" (unsproutable, sterile seed). This makes a difference because sterile seed stays hard and ungerminated amongst its soft and growing "neighbors," sometimes giving you an unpleasant "I-just-bit-down-on-something-hard" surprise in your salad. If you go to the trouble of buying seed labeled "for sprouting" then it will usually also be labeled "organic"—highly desirable because chemicals used on any plant get stored in the seeds, and organic seeds will not be treated with chemicals.

I don't use any one source for my sprouting seed. For sprouts of dried beans and grains I simply use whatever beans and grains I have in the house. I always buy my grains and beans in bulk. Sometimes they are organic and sometimes not, and although they are not specially sorted for sprouting, I don't often get many clinkers in any case. For seed that will make my "green sprouts" such as alfalfa, radish, or sunflower seeds, I buy smaller amounts, perhaps one-half pound to one pound at a time. More likely these seeds will be organic, but not necessarily specially sorted, and again, I don't get many clinkers. I get all of my seed from the health food store or my food-buying co-op. Mail ordering is another way to get excellent sprouting seeds. You can get a high quality and great variety of seeds, along with state-of-the-art instructions and equipment (such as handy growing baskets) from The Sprout House in Great Barrington, Massachusetts (see the Supplies Appendix B).

Check the Bottoms on Store-Bought Sprouts

Many consumers like to get their sprouts ready-to-eat and happily this can happen nowadays at most regular grocery stores as well as health food stores. Some of the most commonly available sprouts at stores are alfalfa, radish, and several sorts of beans both small and large. A health food store would even be likely to be "farming" sunflower sprouts, alfalfa sprouts and wheat grass sprouts, right before your eyes.

When buying sprouts which are already in a package, always turn over the container they are packaged in so that you can check their bottoms for signs of old age and spoilage that can quickly affect the whole batch. Sprouts are often packaged in small, clear plastic boxes with drainage holes in the bottom which help keep them fresh. If the sprouts are packaged in a plastic bag be specially careful in checking them because they will tend to spoil more easily. The sprout roots should be white and smell fresh. and the tops should have two tiny, bright green leaves for the green types. For the non-green types, which are usually the bean sprouts, look for a uniform whitish color and plumpness from end to end. If the sprouted rootlet-end looks wilted, more than just the tip, or the sprouts are tinged with brownish colorations, this could signal old sprouts that will quickly move into the spoiling stage when you get them home. All sprouts should be crisp, plump and lively looking.

How To Sprout—Lalitha's No-Fuss Method

Sprouting your own seed is actually quite easy and space-efficient, but because different types of seeds might need different techniques to optimally sprout them, beginners sometimes get the impression that sprouting might be tricky to learn. It absolutely is not! Sprouting is so easy to learn, and the results are so quick in coming, that after your first experience of luscious sprouts in just a few days with hardly any effort, you'll be hooked forever.

Both Sproutman Steve Meyerowitz's book *Sprouts the Miracle Food!*, and Carol Nostrand's book *Junk Food to Real Food* (see Recommended Bibliography for both) give detailed instructions on several methods of sprouting and the best methods to use with each type of seed. But, for years before I ever read any instructions I had been sprouting whatever I needed by the simple method of soaking seeds in water in a glass jar overnight. My jar was covered with cheesecloth held on by a rubberband. The next morning I would strain off the soak water, refill the jar with fresh water once again and then turn it upside down on my dish rack to drain thoroughly and start germinating while I went off to work. After that I would begin rinsing and draining them thoroughly, twice each day (it took about one minute before and after work), until they got to be the size and quality I wanted. The green leaf ones, like alfalfa and radish, got somewhat green (because, luckily, light shown through the glass jar where it sat on my kitchen counter); the non-chlorophyll sprouts, like lentils and wheat, grew little 1/4-inch to 1/2-inch tails, and then I ate them. If I ever forgot to rinse and drain them for a day or two, sometimes they dried up or rotted on me and sometimes they did not—I think it depended on the season whether my forgetfulness was forgiven or not.

Now I know that my sprouts could have been much greener, juicier, and power-packed if I had been following expert procedures. So, I suggest getting Steve Meyerowitz's *Sprouts the Miracle Food*, or Carol Nostrand's *Junk Food to Real Food*. Their methods are much more efficient, fool-proof and fun—like the sprouting basket and sprouting bag methods along with the clever table-top greenhouses called "Sprout Houses" sold by Sprout House, Inc. Look up Sprouts in the Supplies Appendix B for mail order information on all these sprouting "appliances."

Better Beans

A smart cook will often soak and then sprout all beans intended for cooking as this catalyzes the predigestion of the sprout carbohydrates and other components, making them highly digestible and more nutritious. In practical terms, you simply use the same large, non-aluminum, pot you intend to cook beans in, as a sprouting container for a couple of days. After the initial soaking of a pound or two of beans for several hours in room temperature water, or overnight (they must swell and become fully plump enough to easily poke a fingernail into), rinse them thoroughly, drain them and let them sit in their pot for at least twelve hours. In this time most beans will begin to split open, signaling the beginning of the sprouting process. Don't make the mistake of pouring hot water over the beans to get them to soak and swell faster, as this kills them. They will still swell up but they won't sprout! After sprouting your beans, cook them for several hours as you normally would. For myself, if I plan it right, after I soak a pot of beans overnight I usually leave beans to sit and do their "sprouting thing" for another day and overnight. Then I rinse them again (a good trick for even further enhancing digestibility), throw away the rinse water onto my house plants, and cook the sprouted beans. The more sprouted they are, the better they digest. Sprouted, cooked beans taste uniquely wonderful!

HEALTHY ADDITIONS, ALTERNATIVES, and TRAVELERS TIPS

There are no real Alternatives to sprouts as they are a unique category unto themselves. However, fresh vegetable juice would be a close second and there is more about vegetable juice in the Carrot chapter. Further healthy Additions would be any fresh, raw, vegetables and fruits—especially those of my *10 Essential Foods*.

For those of us who want the health benefits of living foods but find our lifestyle slowing us down in this regard, there is always the choice of buying a "live food" supplement. As I have mentioned in several other chapters, two exceptional choices are:

1. A predominantly organic, raw, flash dried, whole food concentrate called *Phyt-Aloe* and a chewable version for children or adults called *Phyto-Bears*. These are what I personally use and both are sold mail-order through Rejenitec 1-800-867-2563.

2. Tableted, organic, raw, flash dried, whole leaf *Wheat Grass* and *Barley Grass* made by Pines Intl. Inc. and available at health food stores. (See a fuller description of these items in the

Healthy Additions section of the Broccoli chapter and in Supplies Appendix B.)

Travelers could take along a "live food" supplement, or look for a good salad bar. Perhaps you have noticed, as I have, that sprouts have become standard fare at salad bars in many restaurants. Alfalfa sprouts are even showing up as a standard ingredient in some types of sandwiches. So, things are getting better in the eating-out department.

Growing your own sprouts as you travel, as I described in the TASOLE above, is almost always an option. Seeds for sprouting can be found at markets all over the world, even if you have to try unfamiliar beans/seeds at first. For instance, in Nepal, mustard is a major crop so mustard seed for sprouting might be easy to get. While it is a mildly spicy sprout, it is also tasty and fine to eat in smaller amounts. Also, campers can easily grow sprouts as they hike about, as long as they have access to fresh water. (This is easy enough to find while camping at state and federal parks or hiking near water in wilderness areas where the water might be uncontaminated.) In fact, sprouts are a great camp food because the seeds are light to carry around and can be grown as you need them. (Just take one of Sproutman's sprouting bags with you. Rinse it and hang it in a tree at your campsite whenever you stop for the day.)

Another good traveler's choice, as in every chapter, is dehydrated vegetables which can be found at many camp stores and health food stores.

SURVIVAL CHOICE for COMPROMISING CIRCUMSTANCES

For those of you who are new to sprouts and nervous about adding this food to your diet altogether, you can always start with adding one sprout a day to your salad, increasing the "dosage" by one additional sprout per day. In this way you will end up with a sprout eating habit before you know it!

If you are a serious "Survival Case" for any reason, re-read the information about the high-tech vegetable concentrate supplements in the HEALTHY ADDITIONS above.

KIDS LOVE THIS

Certain sprouted-grain breads are almost like cake! Try the sprouted rye with carrot and raisin,or sprouted wheat with carrot and raisin breads, available at your health food store.

Nature's Path *Manna Breads* makes these items, and the one I use most is the sprouted rye (it does not have the typical heavy "rye" flavor at all). I usually find them in the frozen foods section of the health foods store. These breads are thick, sticky and sweet, and they can be eaten plain or spread with butter and/or fruit spread. They can also be sliced (you have to use a wet serrated knife for this), spread with butter (or cream cheese for an occasional special treat), and put under the broiler for a few minutes. Which reminds me of a short TASOLE.

TASOLE: Once when I was leading a camping trip for a group of about ten eleven-year-old boys and girls, I brought along some sprouted rye-carrot-raisin *Manna Bread* for my personal use. One day, Bob, one of the campers, came wandering past me where I sat eating a hunk of this bread spread with butter. He asked me what he could have for a snack and I pointed him to the regular snack box. Then he asked me what I was eating and I told him it was bread made from sprouts but I hadn't brought it for all the campers because I hadn't thought anyone besides me was into eating sprouts. (Bob in particular was quite outspoken about my weird "health foods.") When he pointed out that it didn't look like "regular bread" I agreed. When he continued to stand there without heading for the children's snack box, I told him where my sprout bread and butter was, in case he wanted to try some.

Next thing I knew Bob was raving about "Lalitha's cake" (that's how sweet and sticky this bread is—sprouted grain has a lot of naturally sweet starch). To my surprise I had to start keeping my bread in a new place to prevent it from being all eaten up by the rest of the campers!

Don't miss this recipe:

LENTIL-TOMATO SOUP (serves 4)

2 Tbs. olive oil
1 onion, chopped
2 cloves garlic, minced
5 cups water or stock
2/3 cups lentils [sprouted as above, if desired]
4 small carrots, sliced
2 stalks celery, chopped
3 Tablespoons pure tomato paste
1/4 tsp. thyme
pinch tarragon
chopped parsley for garnish

Warm the olive oil in a large soup pot. Sauté the onion and garlic in the olive oil. Add the water, lentils, thyme and tarragon. Bring the water to a boil, lower the heat and cook, covered, till the lentils are soft (25 to 30 minutes). Add the carrots, celery and tomato paste. Cook till carrots are soft (about 10 minutes) and flavors are blended.

[Note from Lalitha: Don't forget to sprout your beans ahead of time, as I explain in the Better Beans section this chapter. Quick-sprouted lentils would be great for this Lentil-Tomato Soup.]

Recipe from: Nostrand, Carol. *Junk Food to Real Food* (New Caanan, CT: Keats Publishing, 1994, p. 169). Used with permission.

MEDITERRANEAN CHICKEN & FIGS

1/2 cup green bell pepper
1/2 cup red bell pepper
1/2 cup yellow bell pepper
1/2 cup mushrooms, quartered
1/2 cup yellow onion
4 cloves garlic, minced
4 chicken breasts, skinless and boneless
2 Tbs. olive oil
1/4 tsp. coarse black pepper
1/2 Tbs. sea salt, or salt substitute
10 ounces California dried Figs, in bite-sized pieces
1 Tbs. fresh parsley, chopped
1 Tbs. fresh basil, chopped
1/2 cup white wine

Clean and slice vegetables. Cut chicken into strips 2 inch x 1/4 inch. Stir fry chicken strips in olive oil in heavy saucepan over medium heat for 3 minutes. Add all vegetables and seasonings, except Figs, parsley, and basil. Continue to cook for 15 minutes. Add Figs, parsley and basil and mix well. Add wine and continue to cook for another 2 minutes. Serve with your favorite green salad and whole grain rice.
Yield: 6 servings
Each serving contains approximately:
Calories 286, Fat 6.29 g, Dietary Fiber 8.97 g, Carbohydrates 37.1 g, Protein 20.9 g, Sodium 70.5 mg, cholesterol 45.3 mg
Calories from protein: 29%
Calories from carbohydrates: 51%
Calories from fats: 20%

Recipe and nutritional information from: California Fig Advisory Board, 3425 N. First St., Suite 109, Fresno, CA 93726. 1-209-445-5626

13

MEAT, FISH, POULTRY AND DAIRY

ARE NOT ESSENTIAL FOODS. . . BUT CAN BE USED WISELY

Many people are concerned about getting enough protein in their diet and are confused about whether or not they will survive without eating animal products on a daily basis. "How can the *10 Essential Foods* possibly be complete without including some animal foods?" you may ask. In addition, you may have seen health food stores advertising special "organic meats, eggs and milk products" and it has made you wonder what this might imply about the animal products we commonly see at the usual grocery store.

After "digesting" the information about protein in the Almond, Brown Rice, and Sprout chapters, it becomes clear that we can certainly get enough protein from vegetable sources while avoiding the health hazards associated with animal foods. It is obvious that the plant kingdom can cover the "nutritional bases" represented by the animal kingdom, while the animal kingdom cannot cover the "nutritional bases" represented by the plant kingdom. At the same time, animal-source foods *can* be used to support health on those occasions when they are the chosen foods, if you learn some specifics on what to choose, what to avoid, healthy quantities ... and why. Let's start with the story on fish.

FISH FOLLIES

Michael Colgan Ph.D., C.C.N., a responsible researcher and favorite author of mine, is one of a growing number of nutrition experts who fearlessly report the bare facts, without trying to make them "nice" all the time. Dr. Colgan is the author of several books on nutrition and director of the Colgan Institute for Nutritional Science. The following graphic description of the "fish situation" is excerpted from his book *Optimum Sports Nutrition: Your Competitive Edge* (Ronkonkoma, NY: Advanced Research Press, 1993, pp.45-46. Reprinted with permission).

In 1992 Consumer's Union published results of a six-month investigation of the fish industry. They bought fish from the same places you buy it, supermarkets, grocery stores, and specialty fish shops. They sampled seven popular varieties, salmon, flounder, sole, catfish, swordfish, lake whitefish, and clams.

Almost 40% of the fish samples were beginning to spoil at the time of purchase. Ninety percent of the swordfish were contaminated with mercury. Half the whitefish and 40% of the salmon contained polychlorinated biphenyls (PCB's). The clams were laced with arsenic and lead. And this is the one that really got me: almost half of all the fish samples were contaminated with bacteria from *animal or human feces.*

Microbiology experts reported to Consumer's Union that sewage outflows were not the source of fecal contamination of the fin fish, only clams. The fin fish became contaminated **after** [*his emphasis*] being caught. The report cites a litany of appalling sanitary practices during handling, processing, and distribution. Fecal coliform counts above 10 per gram is the standard for contamination. One in five of the Consumer's Union samples had counts *exceeding 100 per gram.* Vomit city!

The American fish industry is a stinking mess. Preliminary results of the Food and Drug Administration's review of 3,852 fish-processing plants released in February 1992, were so bad that, as I write [1993], they are hastily staffing their new Office of Seafood to try to regain control. They would not put a number on it, but they did tell me that the problems would take years to solve. If you are going to use fish as a low-fat source of protein, you have to protect yourself.

Dr. Colgan lists which fish to stay away from altogether. He also lists the contaminated waters—probably most of the ones you and I have ever bought fish from.

He has good words to say about fish from New Zealand, Alaskan, and Australian waters but says that even in Alaskan waters there is now some radioactive waste from defunct Soviet testing sites. The bottom line for best buy was orange roughy from Australasian waters, "virtually contamination free," and flounder and sole (these are primarily from Alaskan waters), "the least contaminated in the Consumer's Union study."

Canned fish, such as tuna, can be a good protein food for those on-the-go, if you are a smart shopper. On this subject Dr. Colgan writes:

> ...canned tuna deserves the last word. There is no bacteria problem because the canning involves high heat that kills everything. But tests by the Consumer's Union showed that 50% of the cans they bought contained filth from insects, rodents, and birds. [*Even though there was a massive clean-up effort in this country for canned fish in 1979 which virtually cleaned canned fish of all filth.*] ... since then, almost all canning has moved outside the US, to countries that have low-low standards of hygiene. [*Back to square one.*] (p. 47)

Dr. Colgan finishes off with saying that the best tuna in the Consumer's Union study was canned albacore (white tuna). He suggests, when buying tuna, to get water-packed tuna canned in this country. His preferred brands were *Bumble Bee*, *Lady Lee*, and *Empress Fancy*. If these brands are not available to you, simply look for another water-packed tuna canned in this country.

MEAT MADNESS

Now that you have the scoop on fish, I've got to tell you that the story is no better for any other type of meat unless it is "organically grown."

Livestock today, from poultry to beef, are subjected to ugly amounts of toxic substances of all sorts, including artificial hormones, growth stimulants, pesticides and antibiotics. Next, their living conditions are so crowded, unsanitary and inhumane, that the spread of disease and parasite infection becomes a frequent horror that calls for dosing the animals with more toxic chemicals, such as additional antibiotics and Toxaphene, to kill the parasites. Toxaphene is so poisonous, writes Humbart Santillo author of *Intuitive Eating* (p. 32), that, "In the most microscopic dose it produces cancer, birth defects, and causes bones to dissolve in lab animals." Dr. Santillo quotes Dr. Adrian Goss, the chief scientist for EPA's Hazards Evaluation Division, as saying: "It is abundantly clear that Toxaphene is an extremely potent carcinogen. I have never encountered an agent purposefully introduced into the environment which has a carcinogenic propensity as clearly marked or as pervasive." Yet, Santillo sums up: "... each year over 1,000,000 cattle are dipped in or sprayed with Toxaphene."

As any health professional or informed consumer should know, poisons are as easily absorbed into an animal's tissues through skin, as through the mouth via feed and medications. (Of course the same is true for us human animals.) Clearly, most animal products contain minute amounts of awful poisons which when ingested accumulate bit by bit in our tissues and organs. By the time a consumer starts noticing a deterioration in immune system health, so much time has passed by, and so much more poison has been accumulated, that our symptoms—from diabetes, to arthritis, to cancer, to chronic infections—are rarely seen to be related to these animal-food sources at all!

The side effects of the continual dosing of meat animals with antibiotics causes them to develop strains of microbes resistant to any treatment. Thus we get strains of salmonella bacteria that end up in the meat we buy and eat, which in turn cause the more than 4,000,000 cases of salmonella poisoning reported each year in the United States. This is true for all non-organic domestic meats, from fowl to beef and everything in between.

Some meat farmers feed their animals with disgusting blends of their own manure, the ground up bodies of fellow meat animals (enforced cannibalism), or sawdust and ammonia to save on "production costs," not caring that the quality of their meat is being compromised to the point of insanity. When some of these facts were revealed by ex-cattleman Howard Lyman, on Oprah Winfrey's show, Oprah responded with, "That is alarming to me! You have just stopped me cold from eating another burger!" The whole story gets worse and worse, but I think you are getting the picture. If you want more details, read the section "Chemicals in Our Foods" in *Intuitive Eating*, or delve into one of the many source materials the author cites.

Another eye-opener book, which is a "must have" resource as far as I am concerned, is *The Safe Shopper's Bible* by David Steinman and Samuel Epstein, M.D.

DAIRY PRODUCTS AND EGGS-STRAVAGANZA

For starters, milk and eggs, being concentrated parts of the reproduction cycle of animals, of necessity and design hold a concentration of substances fed to the animals, for good or ill.

In humans, good nutrition and environmental conditions produce healthy, balanced offspring with body tissues free of disease, while poor nutrition and polluted environments produce all sorts of diseased conditions in mind and body which can be passed on to a gestating fetus, or through mother's milk, mother's ovum, and father's sperm. The same is true for other animals. Humans often unknowingly or uncaringly eat the milk, flesh and eggs of highly-contaminated animals—the very same animals our government agencies pronounce "just fine for eating" and "Grade A." Would a consumer knowingly choose to eat animal products from unhealthy sources? Probably not, but that is just what many of us are doing: perhaps because we think we are "protected by government agencies," and it is too frightening to think about anyway.

The milk, eggs, and fat of an animal, just as in humans, often carry the highest concentrations of antibiotics, hormones, and other chemicals fed or sprayed onto those animals, as I mentioned earlier. These can be just as destructive to human health as they are to the animals who have been forced to ingest them. For instance, I have personally known many cases of women's health being dramatically and adversely affected by the unnatural and concentrated synthetic hormone content in milk, butter, and eggs from animals raised in the common and toxic manner I have described. Likewise, in farming communities I have known of young men who developed characteristics such as female-type breasts as a result of eating lots of eggs and the meat from chickens which were fed large amounts of hormones to increase their production. The bodies of these young men only returned to normal when they followed advice to stop eating the products of their farms! Some of these young men changed to eating "organic" varieties of these same foods without the symptoms of hormone imbalance and ill health returning.

The Health Advisory for Foods in *The Safe Shopper's Bible* (p. 309) says it all:

> Prefer fruits and vegetables over meat and dairy foods, even if you do not have organically grown produce. While non-organic fruits and vegetables are contaminated with pesticides, so are animal foods—even more so. Plant foods, however, also provide vital nutritional content, including beta-carotene (the plant form of vitamin A), vitamin C and fiber; all are extremely important for the prevention of a wide range of diseases, including heart attack and cancer. Meat, poultry and dairy simply cannot duplicate the nutritional benefits of fresh produce, and they also bring a lot of saturated fat into the diet, which is not only bad for your heart and your arteries, but also is where many of the potent and toxic pesticides and industrial chemicals that permeate the food supply concentrate. Best to favor organic produce!

The Milk Myth

There is so much information these days debunking the "drink more milk" myth of our childhoods, that I could not possibly cover it all. I will report a few resources here. Julian Whitaker M.D., author of the well-known *Health and Healing* newsletter and director of the medical clinic, Whitaker Wellness Institute in Newport Beach, CA, wrote a long article about the "dark side of milk" in his March 1996 newsletter (p. 6). He states:

> Chronic ear infections, which plague 20 to 40% of all children under the age of six, are associated with early bottle-feeding with cow's milk, and dairy allergies have been firmly established as the primary cause of such infections.

Commercial milk is the major cause of iron deficiency anemia in babies, and this is why pediatric guidelines now recommend that babies under one year of age not be given cow's milk.

Perhaps the most insidious residue in milk comes from two hormones called "bovine somatotropin" (BST), and "bovine growth hormone" (BGH). These are given to cows to increase their production of milk, which they do, by 10% to 25%. Treated animals, however, have a significantly increased incidence of mastitis, or udder infections, so they are given antibiotics more often, and their milk contains "antibiotic traces," as well as pus and bacteria.

Both Monsanto, the company that makes BST [and BGH] ... and the FDA claim that milk from BST/BGH cows is indistinguishable from regular milk. This is simply not true ...

Dr. Whitaker drives home his point with shocking information about the relationship of BST with tumor growth, together with the "web of deception" that has caused BST to be "sold" to consumers as perfectly safe. The same is true for BGH.

Regarding bovine growth hormone, or BGH, Steinman and Epstein carefully describe the deceptive nature of the FDA's so-called "safe" finding regarding its use. In further substantiation of the Dr. Whitaker report quoted, Steinman and Epstein give a litany of stress diseases such as kidney and heart abnormalities, infertility, and arthritis which are greatly encouraged by the use of growth hormones such as BST and BGH. They go on to describe some of the uninvestigated health hazards to humans associated with the use of these hormones in cows. Apparently, the particular insulin-like growth factors (IGF's) stimulated by, and associated with, BST- and BGH-use in cows for the purpose of artificially increasing production of meat and milk, are suspiciously identical to IGF's found in humans. Since these bovine IGF's can turn up in a treated cow's milk, it is suspected that these insulin-like growth factors in a BST- or BGH-treated cow's milk could induce abnormal growth in infants drinking the milk and promote colon and breast cancers in women.

Hormone-stimulated cows have more infections and must be treated with more antibiotics. Not only do these antibiotics pass into the milk, as I've reported, they also result in the development of stronger strains of bacteria and viruses which are resistant to the original antibiotics. These more virulent agents can also pass into the milk and maybe into the milk-drinkers as well. There is also a good chance that a side effect of growth hormone usage in cows could be an increased stimulation of the release, into the body fat and milk of the cows, of the pesticides and other contaminants present in the animal's food or environment. (This is because of the relationship between the growth hormones and the fat metabolism of the animal.)

The European and Canadian governments have put a ban on the use of these growth hormones, for economic and health reasons, pending more research.

The Safe Shopper's Bible is also unequivocal about the significant health dangers in dairy products, including milk. I will condense (no pun intended) some of the milk data for you; and believe me, I am giving you a short version of this extensive (and often scary) information:

First, the dairy products with the most fat (i.e., butter, ice cream, cheeses, whole milk) are full of toxic amounts of carcinogenic pesticides such as chlordane, DDT and dieldrin. (I know this applies to the fat that comes with all types of meat too.) Secondly, horrific amounts of a variety of antibiotic residues are found in milk. The FDA says that these amounts are "safe levels," but many other expert researchers categorically disagree. (My own observations support this disagreement.) Sulfa drugs and their metabolites, along with drugs such as dioxin and chloramphenicol used with dairy cows, are carcinogenic and make their way into our milk supply. And, the "... FDA's own 1990 screening tests indicate that 46% of all milk samples contained more than one sulfa drug residue," (p. 341). Finally, authors Steinman and Epstein report that milk can contain radioactive contaminants from nuclear plants. Any dairy located near a nuclear plant is "bad news" since short-lived radioactive isotopes can still be present in that milk when it is purchased. Wary consumers should at least find out where their milk comes from.

LALITHA RANTS: Whatdyamean *cows are being forced to intake hormones to increase their milk production to more than their bodies can stand, which makes them so sick they need toxic drugs to stay alive! ... and that pesticides in their food get*

*into their bodies and milk and cause health problems just
like they do in humans!*

*All those "sicko" chemicals then get into the meat and
milk that many of us eat ... and we are supposed to feel
"safe" about it just because the FDA says so, even though
lots of others say "not safe"? Huh? Huh?*

*I don't know about your food store, but at mine, if a
local dairy wants to say on its milk label that this milk is
growth-hormone free, it must also include an FDA-mandat-
ed explanation saying that there is no significant difference
in milk whether cows have been given growth hormones or
not! I've learned that most of the milk on the usual grocery
store shelf is from hormone-stimulated cows unless it says
otherwise! Can you believe it?*

*What do we need all that extra milk for anyway? Are we
short on milk? No way! We have a continual national sur-
plus of milk, for criminny sakes (trying to be polite when
writing a rant is frustrating), and small dairy farms are
going out of business because of it! Who stands to gain by
this giant fiasco? Wellllll ... there is Monsanto and other big
chemical companies who make the hormones, and then of
course the antibiotics to fix the cows with afterwards. Then
there are the big milk distributors and the ... Yikes! I hope
I still have that BGH consumer-information telephone number—oh yeah, it is (202) 466-2823. I'd better catch my
breath, before I give them another call.*

Despite what you might have been educated to believe, there
are not many, if any, good health reasons to drink and eat dairy
products in the first place. In fact, there are a lot of myths floating around about these foods:

- Myth—Drinking milk neutralizes stomach acid.

   Milk can *temporarily* (perhaps for twenty minutes or less)
soothe stomach pain from acidity, but it soon has a rebound
effect and in fact stimulates more stomach acid than you had
to complain about in the first place! Milk is at the top of the
list of foods that *produce* stomach acid. The more milk you
drink (milk is alkaline), the more stomach acid is produced
to offset it. Milk's "ulcer fixing" reputation has been thoroughly debunked all over the world.

- Myth—Milk products have calcium that we need for our health.

  Yes, milk products have lots of calcium and yes, calcium is crucial to good health. The bad news is that most of that needed calcium (plus more, which can be taken from body tissues such as bones), is needed to neutralize the heavy and toxic byproduct of uric acid which comes from the digestion of the high protein content in the milk! (This calcium need applies to the over-consumption of concentrated protein foods in general, which is common with the consumption of animal proteins.) With the consumption of animal products such as milk (and meat), often more calcium is "lost" than absorbed!

  Dr. Humbart Santillo in *Intuitive Eating* (p. 81) states: "If osteoporosis were caused by a deficiency in calcium, how would one explain why the Eskimos, who consume 2000 milligrams of calcium a day, suffer from a high rate of osteoporosis? The answer is simple. They also consume 240-400 grams of protein daily from fish, whale, and walrus." Dr. Michael Colgan in *The New Nutrition* (p. 60) says: "After four decades of milk promotion, osteoporosis has become epidemic. Milk just doesn't do the trick." Dr. Julian Whitaker, in his April 1996 *Health and Healing* newsletter (p. 2) writes: "Stress and too much protein and fat in your diet [*the concentrated fat and protein in milk and other animal products are big offenders here*] make your body acidic ... A more serious consequence of acidity is that it causes calcium to be mobilized out of your bones to buffer the acid and make you more alkaline ... The slightly acidic condition brought on by eating too much protein is a primary reason we have such widespread osteoporosis."

  Plenty of digestible, high-quality calcium, often of equal concentration yet higher availability than in milk, can be gotten from plant sources such as Broccoli, Almonds, Figs and Dulse along with their listed Healthy Additions in *10 Essential Foods*. Interestingly, green foods (those containing chlorophyll) specifically help in recovery from diseases such as arthritis and gout which many of us know are caused by the over-acidity associated with a high-in-animal-protein diet. Green foods, chlorophyll foods, help because they can shift the unhealthy acid state of the body back toward a more healthy alkalinity, while providing an abundance of amazing phytochemicals to facilitate repairs. (For those of you who relate to this and feel you need extra help, check out the list of Green-Foods supplements in my Supplies Appendix B.)

* Myth—Children must have milk to stay healthy. Without it how will they get the calcium and protein they need?
    My answer to the previous myth applies here too. In addition, milk products are one of the top-rated foods offensive to a great many children, as proven in research all over the world. A great variety of chronic and often "mysteriously unexplained" symptoms in children have been traced to the consumption of dairy products (and I bet it applies to adults too). These symptoms include: chronic allergies of all sorts; continual mucous congestion in the intestines, lungs and/or sinuses; migraine headaches with or without epileptic seizures; ear infections; compromised immunity; continual intestinal disturbances such as diarrhea; hyperactivity and skin disturbances. Health investigators attribute these conditions, at least in part, to the fact that, sometime between the ages of eighteen months and four years of age, humans loose the enzyme *lactase*, responsible for the digestion of milk sugar. Also, other milk-product components—such as those grouped as "milk solids," concentrated protein, and fats—are often inadequately digested, resulting in toxic digestive "leftovers" such as the "calcium-gobbling" uric acid I wrote about earlier. A startling quantity and variety of these digestive "leftovers" are not automatically flushed from the body through eliminative channels such as the bowels, kidneys or liver as many of us like to believe. Instead, they are stored in our body tissues, including the organs, and contribute mightily to the above list of complaints.
    Adverse health symptoms often don't appear immediately but build over time until seemingly "unexpected" health symptoms arise to plague us. Commonly a child's adverse health symptom from milk ingestion may not occur until a few hours or days later. Consequently, both parents and doctors find the correspondence hard to believe, until they *eliminate* milk products completely from the child's diet for a week or two. (I have met mom's who think "eliminate" means to cut down on milk products for a day or two. This is not enough to give the body a fair chance to begin to rebalance itself.) Unfortunately, children often love and crave the foods that bring on their worse health symptoms. They

frequently eat large amounts of the offending food and will even fight for it—milk being a common example.

Now for a few facts on the subject:

- Fact—Casein, a substance in cow's milk, is used to make glue.
  There is 300% more casein in cow's milk than in mother's milk. Over time, (for some consumers we are talking no time at all) this casein also *acts like* glue in the human digestive tract, literally coating it and actually slowing down, or stopping, the flow of the nutrients from all our food. Some of us fair better under this sticky, digestion-inhibiting load than others, but there is no reason to put up with it at all, given the many tasty beverage alternatives to milk which I will mention later in the chapter.

- Fact—Diseases implicated with dairy consumption in significant research studies around the world include: arthritis, asthma, prostate cancer, heart disease, high cholesterol, chronic joint pain, ulcers, and osteoporosis. For full details on the osteoporosis and nutrition/milk subject, see *The New Nutrition: Medicine For The Millennium* by Dr. Michael Colgan.

Now, after all this, you may wish to have a source of information that says it all — authoritatively and altogether, in one book! Get the book *Don't Drink Your Milk!* by Frank Oski, M.D., former Chairman, Department of Pediatrics, Johns Hopkins University (Syracuse, N.Y.: Mollica Press, 1983).

Whether you are an occasional consumer of animal products, or someone who "feels the need" every day, you can learn to limit your health risks by educating yourself to choose and handle these products wisely.

FOOD POISONING—LESSEN THE RISK

Most of us have heard of the type of food poisoning commonly called "salmonella poisoning." Salmonella is a highly toxic type of bacteria causing salmonellosis; the acute infection of the gastrointestinal tract, sometimes fatal, characterized by symptoms such as vomiting, diarrhea, nervous system interference, paralysis, etc. Even the cooking of meats is not a guaranteed protection against this bacteria, and the usual antibiotic treatments for salmonella poisoning are becoming steadily less effective as antibiotic-resistant strains of salmonella seem to have evolved faster with the use of the antibiotics!

Salmonella is only one of many human-carried pathogens, which also include other bacteria, and numerous parasites and viruses associated with fresh foods including animal foods such as chicken, eggs, fish, or beef. (Nine different types of salmonella alone are listed in *The Healing Power of Grapefruit Seed*. See Recommended Bibliography.)

So, just as I suggest a disinfecting-detoxfying soak using Grapefruit extract for fruits and vegetables, I also suggest it for meats. Use twenty to forty drops of Grapefruit extract per gallon of water as a soak, or as a spray. For soaking, soak your meats for approximately twenty minutes. See a more detailed explanation of this procedure for disinfecting-detoxifying meats in chapter 2. Grapefruit extract is potent and is used by professional meat-handlers to lessen the spreading of the wide variety of human-carried contaminants I have mentioned.

CHOOSING WISELY: MEAT, FISH, POULTRY, and DAIRY PRODUCTS

Despite all this "bad news" about animal products, I know certain types of people whose health can be positively affected with the *wise* use of animal products in their diet! Even though this idea flies in the face of a great quantity of recent research, and I am no scientist myself, it is apparent to me that, for a particular type of individual (and they are quite in the minority), the consumption of animal products in very small yet regular servings (especially flesh foods as opposed to milk), seems to be crucial to their well-being. Without a little animal-based food (this might be one egg a week, or two to four ounces of meat every day), no matter how cleverly planned their vegetarian diet might be, the health of these people seems to suffer. I have heard many theories about particular factors that make this so, including race, age, environment, climate, mineral balances, fast oxidation versus slow oxidation, alkaline/acid balance, yin/yang, neurosis, you name it! Yet, while these theories make some sense (they each sound so convincing when explained), intuitively I feel they are still off the mark. I am dissatisfied with convenient answers, but I still support the needs of these "mystery types."

To complicate my investigations, there are also those whom I have met who claim to absolutely "need" meat every day, perhaps at every meal, and who I see are obviously ruining their health because of it. These are not the minority-types I am speaking of. The bottom line to these questions of what to eat, when, where, with whom, and whether our health can afford it or not, are all questions each must assess for herself or himself.

Therefore, while I strongly suggest a *highly limited* intake of animal-based foods for the great majority of people, the following principles can help anyone, for any reason, to make the best choices regarding which animal-based foods they include in their diets.

> **Principle #1.** Try to get products from organic sources—from animals that have not been fed, sprayed, or inoculated with all those nasty chemicals. This is becoming easier to do as many health food stores now have meat counters, similar to conventional grocery stores. At a good health food store, the major and crucial difference is that their meat, fish, poultry, eggs, and milk products are all organically farmed.

> **Principle #2.** Choose low-fat or no-fat animal products.

> **Principle #3.** Try eating smaller portions of animal products when you do eat them. Remember what I wrote above, about a high protein and/or fat intake and the negative results to your health. If you want to keep within the suggested range of 25 to 35 grams of protein a day, you can see from the list that follows how it adds up very quickly. Remember, during a given day, in addition to any of the dietary sources of protein listed below, you will also be getting added protein from the grains, nuts, seeds, vegetables and other foods you eat.

Protein Content Sampling
- 1 oz. cooked light meat turkey = 9.3 grams protein
- 1 oz. rump roast = 4.25 grams protein
- 1 oz. chicken breast = 4.6 grams protein
- 1 oz. halibut fish = 6 grams protein
- 1 oz. fresh salmon = 6.3 grams protein
- 1 lg. egg = 6.5 grams protein

- 1 oz. 2% fat cottage cheese, not packed = 2 grams protein
- 1 oz. American cheddar cheese = 7 grams protein
- 1 cup low-fat milk = 8 grams protein

Be careful here. Not many people will only eat two or three ounces of one of these animal products *in a day*. More likely an average consumer would eat more than this at every meal, every day! Even for children, who often need more protein than adults, it is easy to see how this dietary need can easily be abused.

Principle #4. Experiment with not eating animal products every day. This can make a huge and positive difference in your body's ability to more completely utilize those products when you do eat them.

Principle #5. If you need to, buy a milk-digesting enzyme or protein-digesting enzyme supplement at the health food store to use when you are eating animal products. This can immediately help you to digest your food more efficiently and completely, and lessen toxic digestive leftovers. Two brands of digestive supplements that I know work very well are *Prevail* and *Rainbow Light*; found at most health food stores.

Principle #6. Cultured milk products are far and away the best for milk-lovers, so go for the live-culture yogurt without all the additives and sweeteners. (You can add your own sweeteners later). In fact, for those who must have their milk, there is comfort in the fact that the healthy cultures of bacteria in "live" yogurts can enhance immunity, kill off certain unwanted strains of unhealthy bacteria, and increase production of antibodies in our blood (the natural killers of disease organisms). However, if you want the life-enhancing benefits of these yogurt cultures, without the health-degenerative effects of the other properties of milk, you can get help through the use of a broad spectrum, digestive bacteria supplement such as the *Inner Ecology* product of the Prevail company, or the *Symbiotics With FOS* product of the Nutricology company (both at health stores). These give a dramatically wider range of the healthy digestive bacteria than yogurt can offer, without any of the health deficits of milk components as I've described above.

Principle #7. If you are lucky and can get it, buy milk that has not been "double-whammied" with homogenization. Homogenization causes the fat in the milk to bind with the other milk components so they won't separate. But then, those bonded "blobs" won't separate in your digestive track all that well either, and they generally stick in your gut in unhealthy ways. Have you ever wondered why even non-fat milk is homogenized? I bet it's because it prolongs shelf life even more than just plain pasteurization (but don't start me thinking about that one!).

Principle #8. Goat's milk is an excellent alternative to cow's milk because it has a protein density much closer to mother's milk and a more moderate casein content. These traits make goat's milk easier to digest. Many a babe has been saved by drinking goat's milk when mother's milk was not available and cow's milk out of the question, partly because of the things I have disclosed about it above. Although I have heard some friends complain they did not like the "goaty" flavor of goat's milk, I have never had a problem finding a supply that was sweet, mellow, and delicious. Check at a local health food store, and/or call local farmers for leads to a local "goat hobbyist."

Principle #9. For milk alternatives buy rice milk, soy milk, and amazake (a delicious, naturally sweet, high-protein drink with a milk-like consistency, made from sweet Brown Rice). These are all available at health food stores. Or, do like many of my friends do and put pineapple juice on your breakfast cereal! Check out the book *Junk Food to Real Food* by Carol Nostrand. Carol's book not only tells you how to make delicious milk-style beverages out of healthy seeds or whole grains such as Almonds, sesame seed, sunflower seed and Brown Rice, but she gives fantastic, unique and healthy recipes of all sorts besides. (Even recipes for pies and pancakes are included.) Along with this information, Carol tells you how to outfit your kitchen for healthy living in your "food department."

Principle #10. Don't be a fanatic. Who can go through life without ice cream once in a while, or having turkey at Grandmother's Thanksgiving feast? For many people the dilemma of whether or not to eat these foods on rare and special occasions causes unnecessary anxiety and social tangles. Don't get so serious about these things that you make yourself (and perhaps others) sick over them. Lighten up! Just be educated in your choices!

One last recipe:

QUICK FISH FOR ONE

1/4 lb. fillet of flounder or sole
2 Tbs. water
2 Tbs. soy sauce
1 inch fresh raw ginger root, minced

Put the fish in a low Pyrex baking dish. Add enough water and soy sauce and ginger to just barely cover the fish. Put the dish into the broiler and broil approximately 5 minutes. While broiling, spoon some of the liquid mixture over the fish.

Optional: Marinate the fish in the mixture for 1/2 hour before broiling.

Recipe from: Nostrand, Carol. *Junk Food to Real Food* (New Caanan, CT: Keats Publishing, 1994, p. 203). Used with permission.

RECOMMENDED BIBLIOGRAPHY

NUTRITION and HEALTH

Balch, Phyllis A., C.N.C. and James F., M.D. *Prescription for Cooking*. Greenfield, IN: PAB Books, 1987. 610 W. Main, Greenfield, IN 46140.

Balch, Phyllis A., C.N.C. and James F., M.D. *Prescription for Nutritional Healing*. Garden City Park, NY: Avery Publishing, 1990.

Beutler, Jade. *Flax for Life*. Encinitas, CA: Progressive Health Publishers, 1996. Available through Barlean's Oils, 1-800-445-3529.

Beutler, Jade and Murray, Michael T., N.D. *Understanding Fats and Oils: Your Guide to Healing with Essential Fatty Acids*. Encinitas, CA: Progressive Health Publishers, 1996. Available through Barlean's Oils, 1-800-445-3529.

Blonz, Edward R., PhD. *The Really Simple No Nonsense Nutrition Guide*. Berkeley, CA: Conari Press, 1993. 1144 65th St., Suite B, Emeryville, CA 94608.

Budwig, Johanna M.D., PhD. *Flax Oil as a True Aid Against Arthritis, Heart Infarction, Cancer, and other Diseases*. Vancouver: Apple Publishing, 1992. Available through Barlean's Oils, 1-800-445-3529.

Budwig, Johanna M.D., PhD. *The Oil Protein Diet*. Vancouver: Apple Publishing, 1992. Available through Barlean's Oils, 1-800-445-3529.

Carper, Jean. *Food Your Miracle Medicine*. New York, NY: Harper Collins, 1993.

Colgan, Dr. Michael, *Optimum Sports Nutrition: Your Competitive Edge*. Ronkonkoma, NY: Advanced Research Press, 1993. (516) 467-3140.

Colgan, Dr. Michael, *The New Nutrition: Medicine for the Millennium*. Ronkonkoma, NY: Advanced Research Press, 1994. (516) 467-3140.

Cooper, Kenneth H., M.D. *Antioxidant Revolution*. Nashville, TN: Thomas Nelson Publishers, 1994.

Dean, Ward, M.D. and Morgenthaler, John. *Smart Drugs and Nutrients*. Menlo Park, CA: Health Freedom Publications, 1991. P.O. Box 2515, Menlo Park, CA, 94026. (415) 321-2374.

Dean, Ward, M.D. and Morgenthaler, John. *Smart Drugs and Nutrients II*. Menlo Park, CA: Health Freedom Publications, 1993. P.O. Box 2515, Menlo Park, CA, 94026. (415) 321-2374.

Duke, James, Ph.D. and Associates. *Phytochemical and Ethnobotanical Database*, National Germplasm Resources Laboratory U.S.D.A., Agricultural Research Service. Available through Internet address: http://www.ars-grin.gov/~ngrlsb/

Erdmann, Robert, PhD. and Jones, Meirion. *Fats That Can Save Your Life*. Encinitas, CA: Progressive Health Publishing, 1995. Available through Bio-Science, (206) 871-6115.

Fischer, William L. *How To Fight Cancer and Win*. Canfield, OH: Fischer Publishing Corp., 1994. (216) 533-1232.

Fryer, Lee and Simmons, Dick. *Food Power From the Sea*. New York, NY: Mason/Charter, 1977.

Gerson, Max, M.D. *A Cancer Therapy: Results of 50 Cases and the Cure of Advanced Cancer by Diet Therapy*. Barrytown, NY: Station Hill Press, 1990.

Jensen, Bernard, D.C. *Chlorophyll Magic From Living Plant Life.* Escondido, CA: Dr. Bernard Jensen, 1981. RT. 1, Box 52, Escondido, CA 92025.

Margen, Sheldon, M.D. and the Editors of the University of California at Berkeley "Wellness Newsletter." *The Wellness Encyclopedia of Food and Nutrition.* New York, NY: Rebus Press (Random House), 1992.

Meyerowitz, Steve. *Sprouts the Miracle Food!* Great Barrington, MA: The Sprout House Inc., 1997. P.O. Box 1100, Great Barrington, MA 01230. 1-800-SPROUTS. E-mail address is: sprout@sproutman.com.

Murray, Michael T., N.D. *Healing Power of Foods.* Roseville, CA: Prima Pubs., 1993. (916) 786-0426.

Murray, Michael T., N.D. *Encyclopedia of Natural Medicine.* Roseville, CA: Prima Pubs., 1990. (916) 786-0426.

Nostrand, Carol. *Junk Food to Real Food.* New Caanan, CT: Keats Publishing, 1994. P.O. Box 876, New Caanan, CT 06840. 1-800-858-7014.

Nutrition Almanac. Nutrition Research, Inc., McGraw-Hill, 1984. (Nutritional data used with permission of the McGraw-Hill companies.)

Oski, Frank, M.D. *Don't Drink Your Milk.* Syracuse, NY: Mollica Press, 1983.

Poisson, Leandre and Gretchen. *Solar Gardening.* White River Junction, VT: Chelsea Publishing Company, 1994.

Santillo, Humbart, N.D. *Food Enzymes: The Missing Link to Radiant Health.* Prescott, AZ: Hohm Press, 1987. P.O. Box 2501, Prescott, AZ 86302. 1-800-381-2700.

Santillo, Humbart "Smokey," N.D. *Intuitive Eating.* Prescott, AZ: Hohm Press, 1993. 1-800-381-2700.

Schauss, Alexander, PhD. *Minerals, Trace Elements and Human Health.* Tacoma, WA: Life Sciences Press, 1996. P.O. Box 1174, Tacoma, WA 98401. (206) 922-0442, FAX (206) 922-0479. To purchase send $12.50, postage included.

Schauss, Alexander, PhD. *The Role of Essential Trace Elements In Human Health and Behavior;* audio cassette tape of his wonderful July 1994 lecture at the National Nutritional Foods Association. Available from Tree Farm Cassetes, 1-800-468-0464.

Seibold, Ronald, M.S. *Cereal Grass, What's In It For You!*. Lawrence, KS: Wilderness Community Education Foundation, 1990. P.O. Box 1261, Lawrence, KS 66044-8261.

Sharamon, Sheila and Baginski, Bodo J. *The Healing Power of Grapefruit Seed*. Twin Lakes, WI: Lotus Light Publications, 1996. 1-800-548-3824.

Steinman, David and Epstein, Samuel S., M.D. *The Safe Shopper's Bible: A Consumer's Guide to Nontoxic Household Products, Cosmetics, and Food*. New York, NY: Macmillan, 1995.

Teas, Jane. *The Consumption of Seaweed as a Protective Factor in the Etiology of Breast Cancer*. Boston, MA: Harvard School of Public Health, 1981. 865 Huntington Avenue, Boston, MA 02115 [Medical Hypotheses, 7(5): 601-603.] Also available through Maine Coast Sea Vegetable Company, (207) 565-2907.

United States Department of Agriculture (USDA). *Human Nutrition Information Service*. 6505 Belcrest Road, Hyattsville, MD 20782. Write to this address for all sorts of new pamphlets on nutrition, including *The Food Guide Pyramid*, (Home and Garden bulletin number 252). Or, get in touch with your own local USDA extension service.

Wallach, Joel, D.V.M., N.D. *Rare Earth: Forbidden Cures*. New Vision independent associate, 1-800-250-8171.

Whitaker, Dr. Julian, M.D. *Health and Healing Newsletter*. Potomac, MD: Phillips Publishing. 1-800-705-5559.

COOK BOOKS

Bradford, Peter and Montse. *Cooking With Sea Vegetables*. New York, NY: Thorsons Publishers, 1986.

Bragg, Paul C., N.D., Ph.D. and Bragg, Patricia, N.D., Ph.D. *Apple Cider Vinegar Health System, Salt-Free Sauerkraut Cook Book*, and others. Santa Barbara, CA: Health Science, 1-800-446-1990.

California Fig Advisory Board, 3425 N. First St., Suite 109, Fresno, CA 93726. (209) 445-5626 (Call them for free fig-information and recipes using figs.)

Esko, Wendy and Edward. *Macrobiotic Cooking for Everyone.* Tokyo, Japan: Japan Publications, 1984. Available at bookstores or from Kushi Institute at (413) 623-5741.

Katzen, Mollie. *Moosewood Cookbook.* Berkeley, CA: Tenspeed Press, 1977. A new, shortened version, is now also available. *Moosewood Cookbook Classics,* 1996.

Katzen, Mollie. *The Enchanted Broccoli Forest.* Berkeley, CA: Tenspeed Press, 1982.

Lewallen, John and Eleanor. *Sea Vegetable Gourmet Cookbook and Wildcrafter's Guide.* Mendocino, CA: Mendocino Sea Vegetable Company, 1995. P.O. Box 1265, Mendocino, CA 95460. (707) 937-2050.

Maine Coast Sea Vegetable Recipes. Franklin, ME: Maine Coast Sea Vegetable Company, 1996. (207) 565-2907. E-mail: mcsv@acadia.net (for lots of great information).

Nostrand, Carol. *Junk Food to Real Food.* New Caanan, CT: Keats Publishing, 1994. P.O. Box 876, New Caanan, CT 06840. 1-800-858-7014.

APPENDIX A

CLINICS

These Clinics incorporate nutritional therapies with state-of-the art allopathic and naturopathic disciplines. Renowned for extraordinary results.:

Atkins Center for Complimentary Medicine. Treats all Diseases. Dr. Robert Atkins, M.D., on 55th Street, New York, NY. 1-800-845-3072.

Burzynski Clinic. Specializes in cancer and treats other illness. Dr. Stanislaw Burzynski, M.D., 12000 Richmond Ave., Suite 260, Houston, TX 77082-2431. (713) 597-0111. Through Dr. Julian Whitaker's *Health and Healing* newsletter, I have been keeping up on the truly extraordinary positive results happening here with curing cancer. At the moment the FDA is trying to give them many problems. In my opinion, this makes them even more highly recommended.

The Kushi Institute. For eighteen years the Kushi Institute has offered programs on the macrobiotic way of life, a natural, whole-foods diet, and a lifestyle that supports vibrant health. Help for serious illness, including cancer, as well as lifestyle education for the prevention of illness. P.O. Box 7, Becket, MA 01223-0007. (413) 623-5741. Check out their web site on the internet at http://www.macrobiotics.org.

Schools of Naturopathic Medicine: In addition to the clinics listed above, there are four highly regarded, accredited, schools of naturopatic medicine in the United States and Canada. These schools have their own clinics and/or can refer people to licensed naturopaths throughout the country. They are: Bastyr University (Seattle WA), National College of Naturopathic Medicine (Portland, OR), Southwest College of Naturopathic Medicine (Tempe AZ) and the Canadian College of Naturopathic Medicine (Toronto, ONT, Canada).

Tijuana, Mexico Clinics. In Tijuana, Mexico, there are many different clinics treating all illness especially cancer. Often they are run by medical doctors from the United States whose therapies were proving successful yet were being forbidden by the FDA. See the book *Tijuana Clinics*, by Sally Wolper from Promotion Publishing, 1-800-231-1776.

Whitaker Wellness Institute. Does not treat cancer, but does handle all else. Julian Whitaker, M.D., 4321 Birch St., Suite 100, Newport Beach, CA 92660. (714) 851-1550.

APPENDIX B

SUPPLIES, RECOMMENDED PRODUCTS and HEALTH ACCESSORIES

This Appendix represents some of the "best finds" from my research and experimentation over many years; my own personal preferences for particular brands of a wide variety of products, including digestive enzymes, Flaxseed oils, condiments, or appliances for the kitchen. Of course, many other great choices can be found at health food stores, groceries, through mail order, etc. and these may suit you better. This list is meant to help get you started and to help you find the products I mention in this book.

The double asterisk (**) next to a product means it is a special favorite of mine that I probably use just about every day. Telephone numbers are provided so that you can contact the companies listed to find out where to buy the products if you can't easily find them (unlikely); or to get information to pass along to your local store to have them start carrying a particular product for you.

CODE EXPLANATIONS:
      H = available at health food stores.
      G = available at many grocery stores.
      M = available by mail order.
      ** = Lalitha's special favorite

APPLIANCES:

CHAMPION JUICER: Plastaket Manufacturing Company Inc., Lodi, CA. For the consumer that wants a tough, fairly efficient and easy to clean fruit and vegetable juicer while investing a more modest sum than is called for with the two following machines, I suggest the Champion Juicer. I have been using mine for years with never a problem and it looks like it will never quit! They cost about $275. Call Albion Distributors 1-800-247-1475, or check your local health food store. (H, M).

GREEN POWER JUICE EXTRACTOR: Green Power International, Downey, CA. As far as vegetable juice extractors go, this one is the "newest and bestest" on the market — an upscale in juicer technology. It is tough, easy to clean, efficient and handles many other food preparation jobs. When I saw this "cadillac juicer" at a trade show I was very impressed that it was also very quiet. A big improvement over other machines available. It is also the most expensive (about $600) but will last forever. Call toll free to order one at 1-888-254-7336. (H,M).

VITA-MIX: Vita-Mix,Cleveland OH. This amazing machine is a whole foods juicer — meaning it leaves all the fiber of the whole food in the juice, whereas a juice extractor extracts the juice from the fiber. This machine can take the place of a vegetable juicer, blender, grain grinder and frozen dessert maker! It does all this while maintaining the optimal nutritional content of the whole foods used. It is built to last a lifetime and costs in the $450 range. A real health investment. This company has excellent resource materials on whole foods nutrition, so call them. 1-800-848-2649 (H, M).

FOOD PRODUCTS and HEALTH SUPPLEMENTS:

ARIZONA NATURALS: (see GARLIC)

BEE POLLEN: CC POLLEN COMPANY, Phoenix, AZ. My first choice source for bee pollen. Ask for *High-Desert® Pollen*. This company also carries a high quality *Royal Jelly*.

Many companies claim their pollen is the best, yet I sure don't get the same results with others as I do with CC Pollen brand. Bee Pollen has just about every nutrient known to be essential to human well-being—vitamins, minerals, amino acids, phytochemicals, etc., and much has been written about its health benefits. Bee pollen is a great supplement for most children. It tastes great sprinkled onto breakfast cereal and other foods.

Royal Jelly is the "nectar of the Gods," produced by the Queen honeybee. It is known for its ability to enhance and rejuvenate the body's immune system, thereby reducing the effects of aging. It also contains a concentrated complex of vitamins, minerals and trace elements.

Call the company for interesting literature. 1-800-875-0096 (H, M).

BARLEAN'S ORGANIC OIL: (see OIL—FLAXSEED OIL)

BLUE GREEN ALGAE: (see SUPER FOODS)

BRAGG'S LIQUID AMINOS: Bragg Live Food Products, Santa Barbara, CA. Source for a high protein (in the form of amino acids), brown, liquid, naturally salty-tasting (no salt added), soy-based condiment. No preservatives, not fermented, no alcohol. *Bragg's* has a fantastic taste, which I like much better than soy sauce or tamari. I use *Bragg's* every day, sprinkled onto foods, especially whole grains. This company has several other great products such as unpasteurized apple cider vinegar and books on health, longevity, self-improvement and how to make your own salt-free sauerkraut! 1-800-446-1990 (H).

BROWN RICE:
ARROWHEAD MILLS: Hereford, TX. This fine company provides a huge variety of whole grains, including Brown Rice. They also manufacture some nutritious ready-made breakfast cereals, baking mixes and many other products. In general, Arrowhead Mills is a brand you can trust, but don't give up reading labels on prepared foods. 1-800-858-4308 (G, H).
LUNDBERG FAMILY FARMS: Richvale, CA. A superb source for a great variety of whole grain brown rices. This family-run farm is partly organic (their most expensive rice) and partly "Nutra-Farmed," which is quite close to being organic but not certified organic (and it is less expensive). All their products are of the highest quality.

They make an excellent line of rice cakes too. (916) 882-4551 (H, G, M).

OTHER GOOD BRANDS for Brown Rice and other whole grains in all shapes and forms: Bob's Red Mills, Eden Foods, Texmati Rice and Heartland Mills. (H).

CALCIUM: Calcium is an important mineral supplement for many people, especially those at high risk for, or dealing actively with, osteoporosis. The best supplements I have found, which also contain the synergistic nutrients for calcium maintenance and absorption are:

Bone Builder from Ethical Nutrients/Metagenics (H, M) (1-800-692-9400)

This one has more than 200 studies supporting its use for bone degenerative related conditions and diseases.

Ultra-Cal Night from Source Naturals (H)

Everyday Calcium from Rainbow Light (H)

Complete Calcium from Trace Minerals Research (H)

CC POLLEN: (see BEE POLLEN)

CHLORELLA: (see GREEN FOODS—BLUE GREEN ALGAE)

CITRUS PECTIN: (see GRAPEFRUIT EXTRACT PRODUCTS)

CONCENTRATED FOOD SUPPLEMENTS: (see SUPER FOODS)

CONDIMENTS:
Lalitha's Recommended Condiments:

The following list of condiments are all health-positive additions that may enhance the *10 Essential Foods*. These condiments have all been "tested" by me and many of my friends, and this list represents the ones that have received the high ratings by children as well as adults.

Each condiment listed here is explained elsewhere in this alphabetical Appendix. Just look up the product name, like *Quick Sip* or *Bragg's*, or the generic names, like Mayonnaise or Honey.

All of these condiments should be available at health food stores.

- **BRAGG'S LIQUID AMINOS*
- FLAXSEED LIGNANS WITH MISO: (see recipe in Flaxseeed Oil chapter. Also see OIL and MISO.)
- GINGER PICKLES: (see PICKLES)
- HONEY
- JAMS and JELLIES
- SALSA or HOT SAUCE: (see SALSA)
- MAYONNAISE
- MISO
- MOLASSES
- MUSTARD
- PICKLES
- **QUICK SIP*
- SALSA
- SAUERKRAUT: (see PICKLES)
- SEA PICKLES: (see SEA VEGETABLES)
- SEA SEASONINGS
- UMEBOSHI PLUM PASTE
- VINEGAR

DIGESTIVE ENZYMES: (see ENZYMES)

ECOGENICS: (see GRAPEFRUIT EXTRACT PRODUCTS—CITRUS PECTIN)

EDEN FOODS Inc.: Clinton, MI. An excellent brand for miso (see MISO); sea vegetables of all sorts; and Umeboshi Plum Paste (pickled umeboshi plums). Umeboshi Plum Paste is a salty-sour condiment I truly love. This paste is an excellent digestive aid besides having great flavor. Eden Foods makes hundreds of fine products. 1-800-248-0301 (G, H).

ENZYMES:
PREVAIL INC., Gresham, OR. Source for excellent plant-source digestive enzymes that work on a full spectrum of food components such as fats, carbohydrates, proteins, milk products, fiber, etc. I have personally done experiments with several different digestive enzyme supplement samples. Prevail does a great job—no question. 1-800-248-0885 (H).
RAINBOW LIGHT NUTRITIONAL SYSTEMS INC., Santa Cruz, CA. Top-notch brand of high quality, plant-source digestive enzymes. 1-800-635-1233 (H).

FIBER GREENS PLUS: (see GREEN-FOODS)

FLAXSEED OIL: (see OIL)

GARLIC: Three highly therapeutic brands to try are *Wakanuga, Kwai,* and *Arizona Naturals.* Daily use of garlic will lower blood pressure, lower cholesterol, build immunity, fight infection and build stamina against stress. There is an entire chapter about this amazing food/herb in my book *10 Essential Herbs* (Prescott, AZ: Hohm Press, 1992). All of the listed brands are dependable, and are found at most health food stores. There is a separate listing for Wakanuga, Inc. in this Appendix (G,H).

GINGER PICKLES: (see EDEN FOODS)

GRAPEFRUIT EXTRACT PRODUCTS:
CITRUS PECTIN: One source for this health-helper talked about in the Grapefruit chapter is Ecogenics. A five-week supply will cost approximately $100. 1-800-308-5518 (M) Another source is Allergy Research Group/Nutricology Inc. A four-week supply is approximately $150. 1-800-545-9960 (H).
NUTRIBIOTIC® INC.: Lakeport, CA. Source for grapefruit extract called *Nutribiotic®*, used for the food Detoxifying Process I describe in chapter 2. I value this extract for its health protective qualities when taken internally as well as for its external uses. I never travel without it. They also make the *Non-Soap,* mentioned in chapter 2, which includes grapefruit extract. 1-800-225-4345 (H, M).

GREEN-FOODS:
**KLAMATH BLUE GREEN ALGAE*: This whole food supplement is harvested from Klamath Lake, by Klamath Blue Green, Inc., Mt. Shasta, CA. It is primarily packaged in tablets or powder (those are the forms I use), but the company has just introduced some interesting new blue green algae products such as energy bar snacks.

Blue green algae is a source of protein, B vitamins including B_{12}, beta carotene, and much else. I find it works as a catalyst to many health and healing processes.

The Klamath company does constant and extensive testing of their products for contaminants, and goes to the extra expense of packaging their product in glass to provide extraordinary protection to the beta carotene content. I use it every day. 1-800-327-1956 (H).

Although *Klamath Blue Green Algae* is my favorite type of algae supplement, Spirulina and Chlorella are two other types of algae that have proven highly useful to many consumers, sometimes preferable to Blue Green.

FIBER GREENS PLUS.: A source for this super Green-Food supplement is Healthy Directions. The *Plus* means that, in addition to a concentrated, chlorophyll-rich, green juice, *Fiber Greens Plus* also contains healthy fiber, friendly digestive bacteria, and a special food (called FOS for short) to feed the healthy bacteria into an invigorating colony within you. Recommended by many health professionals—Dr. Julian Whitaker and myself included. 1-800-722-8008 (H, M).

KYROGREEN: Wakanuga of America, Mission Viejo, CA is a source for this quick-mixing, super, Green-Food supplement powder. They also make other potent health products such as their *Kyolic* garlic concentrates. 1-800-421-2998 (H).

PRO-GREENS: Allergy Research Group/Nutricology, Inc., San Leandro, CA is a source of this whole-food supplement. This one is full of several different types of algae and Green Foods, as well as the synergistic components to greatly enhance their health and healing action, including friendly intestinal bacteria. This company's products are always as pure as they say they are. Some of the best product-formulators in the industry work for them and their reputation is the highest. They also sell the "Citrus Pectin" talked about in the Grapefruit chapter. 1-800-545-9960 (H, M).

WHEAT GRASS AND WHOLE LEAF BARLEY GRASS: Pines International, Inc., Lawrence, KS, is a source for these pure, organic, high-quality supplement tablets or powder. A convenient way to get concentrated "green" (chlorophyll) and many other raw food benefits into your diet, no matter what your lifestyle. 1-800-697-4637 (H, M).

HEALTHY DIRECTIONS: (see GREENFOODS—FIBER GREEN PLUS and MAIL ORDER)

HONEY: (Also see MOLASSES) Honey is a food item which must be raw, unheated and unfiltered to have the full health and healing properties for which it is famous. Raw honey has trace minerals, active enzymes, small amounts of pollen, and natural health-positive sugars along with other health-giving properties. Use as a sweetener in place of processed sugars such as corn syrup, sugar cane, etc. I find honey to be such an important health tool that I wrote an entire Appendix about it in my book *10 Essential Herbs*. If the honey you buy is clear and quite thin, it is probably highly heated and filtered during processing; therefore, its health and healing properties are greatly lessened. Health food stores tend to have better quality honey, but I have found an excellent Arizona-grown brand *(Mrs. Crockett's)* at my local supermarket at a great price. Check at your usual food market too. Read the labels; look for any of the words: "raw," "unheated," or "unfiltered." (G, H).

JAMS and JELLIES: The usual sugar-filled jams, jellies and preserves can now be replaced by naturally-sweet and delectable "fruit spreads." These are simply fruits prepared without the processed sugar, preservatives, artificial colorings and flavorings common to the more traditional, commercially prepared products. "Fruit spreads" are still high in sugars, albeit natural fruit sugars, which are less offensive to health. They should not, of course, make up a major portion of one's diet. However, as a condiment for occasional use ... yum! Look for Polaner's brand at regular grocery stores. At health food stores you will find Polaner's as well as Cascadian Farms and R.W. Knudsen. (G, H).

JUICERS: (see APPLIANCES)

KLAMATH BLUE GREEN ALGAE: (see GREEN-FOODS—BLUE GREEN ALGAE)

KWAI, INC.: (see GARLIC)

KYROGREEN: (see GREEN-FOODS—KYROGREEN)

MAIL ORDER: Here are a few mail order sources for high quality Vitamins and other Supplements of all types, including Super-Foods, etc.:

Bragg's Products, Santa Barbara, CA 1-800-446-1990
Healthy Directions, Kearneysville, WV 1-800-722-8008
Home Health, Virginia Beach, VA 1-800-284-9123
Mannatech Inc. (Independent Assoc.) 1-800-820-8510
Nature's Distributors, Fountain Hills, AZ 1-800-624-7114

Nutrition Warehouse, Mineola, NY 1-800-645-2929
Swanson Health Products, Fargo, ND 1-800-437-4148
Vitamin Research Products, Inc., Carson City, NV 1-800-877-24447

MAINE COAST SEA VEGETABLES: Franklin, ME. A source for organically-certified dulse and other Atlantic coast sea vegetables. Their offerings include other sea-vegetable products such as *Sea Seasonings* and *Sea Pickles*, along with an enticing and easy-to-follow cookbook for sea vegetables (see the Cookbooks in the Recommended Bibliography). Buy their products at your health food store, or order products and cookbook via telephone (207) 565-2907 or E-mail: mcsv@acadia.net (H, M). (Also see EDEN FOODS)

MAYONNAISE: When buying mayonnaise look for those made with cold-pressed canola oil. I use Spectrum Naturals brand. Also Hain's brand is reliable. Another worthwhile choice would be cold-pressed safflower oil mayonaise; but only if it is organic. (G, H).

MINERALS: *Concentrace© Low Sodium Trace Mineral Drops*, Trace Minerals Research Inc.This company manufactures and distributes liquid or tableted, full-range, unflavored ionic trace minerals concentrate. Add to water or other beverages or foods. I use these every day. This company also formulates excellent major mineral supplements. Also look under the Calcium listing above and see the Dulse chapter for more information about minerals and the forms they come in. Available at health food stores, or call 1-800-624-7145 for where to buy these minerals near you. (H, M)

MISO: A fermented soybean paste, or soybean plus grain paste—such as rice or barley miso. High in nutrition, and flavorful, as miso contains the salt used in processing. Used in soups, broth, and as a side condiment (use a small bit with a bite of food). I mention miso in the Dulse chapter under Shopping For Sea Vegetables and Other Food Skills. Buy unpasteurized miso, when possible; I always buy Miso Master brand. Another trusty brand is Eden Foods which has pasteurized as well as unpasteurized types. Be sure to check the labels carefully if you are looking for unpasteurized. Unpasteurized miso should be found in the refrigerator of a health store. Also, don't go overboard on the so-called "mellow-miso's." These are not nearly as health-positive as the red or darker ones, partly because they are usually made from other than whole grains (for instance, white rice may be used as a major ingredient). Mellow misos or light misos can also have added sweeteners. (Also see MISO MASTER, and EDEN FOODS) (G, H).

MISO MASTER®: Rutherfordton, NC. Unpasteurized miso of many varieties are available from this company (also known as the American Miso Company). I couldn't find a toll-free telephone number for them but the Miso Master® brand is available at most health food stores. This is absolutely my favorite miso, out of several other brands I have tried. My favorite variety is the *Traditional Red*. (Also see MISO) (H)

MOLASSES: Can be an excellent sweetener! Be certain to buy unsulphured molasses, whether of the light or dark varieties. Unsulphured molasses, especially unsulphured blackstrap molasses, is high in powerful nutrients such as trace minerals, B vitamins, calcium, phosphorus and iron. And molasses has only 42 calories per tablespoon! There are several adequate brands at regular supermarkets as well as at health food stores. (G, H).

MUSTARD: Look for mustards that have no added sugar, colorings, artificial flavorings and preservatives. It is surprising what some manufacturers can do to "ruin" a simple item like mustard. At regular grocery stores, I have found *Grey Poupon* to be tasty and reliable, and at health food stores I tend to buy the Westbrae brand, although there are other tried and true mustards in both locations. (G, H).

NUTRIBIOTIC®: (see GRAPEFRUIT EXTRACT PRODUCTS)

NUTRICOLOGY: (see GREEN-FOODS—PRO GREENS)

OIL:
 **FLAXSEED OIL: Barlean's Organic Oils, Ferndale, WA. Source for best-tasting Faxseed oil. No others compare. 1-800-445-3529 (H).

SPECTRUM NATURAL OILS: Petaluma, CA. A reputable brand for a wide variety of organic, cold-pressed, unrefined or mildly-processed food oils. (707) 778-8900 (G, H).

**PAPAYA JOHNS ENERGY BARS:* (see 10 Essential Snacks Appendix C)

**PHYT-ALOE:* (see REJENITEC)

**PHYTO-BEARS:* (see REJENITEC)

PICKLES: Pickled vegetables are often a favorite with all age groups, and they can be a health aid if you are a smart shopper. Whether you are buying cucumber pickles, sauerkraut, pickled garlic, or a pickled vegetable combination, buy pickled vegetables that contain as little salt (or no salt) as possible and do not buy pickles that contain artificial colorings and flavorings, nor added processed-sugar sweeteners (honey is OK). I have never found such a pickle at a regular grocery store, but health food stores have some luscious brands. Top on my list is Cosmic brand. They manufacture *Cosmic Cukes* and *Cosmic Cabbage* (sauerkraut). Other trustworthy brands are Cascadian Farms and New Morning. To make your own salt-free saurkraut get the *Salt-Free Health Sauerkraut Cook Book* from the Bragg's company at 1-800-446-1990. (Also see SEA PICKLES and VINEGAR) (G, H).

PINES INTERNATIONAL, Inc.: (see GREEN-FOODS— WHEAT GRASS AND BARLEY GRASS)

PREVAIL, INC.: (see ENZYMES)

PRO-GREENS: (see GREEN-FOODS)

**QUICK SIP*: Dr. Bernard Jensen's Hidden Valley Mills, Solana Beach, CA. Another salty-tasting (but no salt added) liquid condiment for sprinkling on foods, but with a different flavor than *Bragg's Liquid Aminos* (also see). You may want to try both to see which one you perefer. *Quick Sip* looks similar to soy sauce but is much better for you nutritionally. I find it has a more appealing flavor than soy sauce. (619) 755-4027 (H)

RAINBOW LIGHT NUTRITIONAL SYSTEMS, INC.: (see ENZYMES)

**REJENITEC: Tacoma, WA. Source for super-foods called *Phytobears* (chewable form for adults and children) and *Phyt-Aloe* (same super-food in capsule form). These are a primarily organic, raw, flash-dried, whole foods concentrate which contain the phytochemical and nutritional equivalent of 8 ounces of fresh-squeezed plant juice in one *Phyt-Aloe* capsule, or 4 ounces of fresh-squeezed plant juice in one chewable *Phyto-Bear*. This super-food is composed of nine different vegetables, several of which are among the *10 Essential Foods*, and three different fruits. This power-packed product retains over 90% of the phytochemicals and over 80% of all the vitamins, minerals, plant digestive enzymes, and soluble fiber from the source fruits and vegetables. The chewable, fruit-sugar sweetened, pure gelatin *Phyto-Bears* (they look similar to the *Gummi Bear®* candy) taste so great that children will fight you for more! I use these products and I love the results! This company also sells other highly effective, immune-supportive products. 1-800-867-2563; FAX (206) 564-9394 (M).

RICE: (see BROWN RICE)

ROYAL JELLY: (see BEE POLLEN—CC POLLEN CO.)

SALSA and **HOT SAUCE:** At grocery stores buy Pace salsa and Crystal hot sauce. These have few if any harmful additives. There are other good brands on the market, but you must be an informed label-reader. Health food stores often stock several commercial brands, and occasionally some local home-made organic salsas. (G, H).

SALT REPLACEMENTS/ALTERNATIVES: (see BRAGG'S, QUICK SIP, MISO and SEA SEASONINGS)

SAUERKRAUT: (see PICKLES)

SEA PICKLES: (see SEA VEGETABLES)

SEA SEASONINGS: Made by Maine Coast Sea Vegetables. These prepared seasonings are recommended as salt replacements as well as for adding spice to your food in general.

They incorporate tasty mixtures of ground sea vegetables, herbs and spices into their formulas. Varieties such as *Dulse with Garlic* appeal to most tastebuds. (Also see MAINE COAST SEA VEGETABLES and EDEN FOODS.) (H, M)

SEA VEGETABLES: (see EDEN FOODS, Inc. and MAINE COAST SEA VEGETABLES)

SEA PICKLES: Pickled kelp, made by Maine Coast Sea Vegetables. Delicious! Give them a try. Buy them at your health food store or direct from Maine Coast Sea Vegetables (see MAINE COAST SEA VEGETABLES above for information). (H, M).

SNACKS: (see the 10 ESSENTIAL SNACKS, APPENDIX C)

SPECTRUM OIL: (see OIL)

SPIRULINA: (see GREEN-FOODS—BLUE GREEN ALGAE)

SPROUT HOUSE, INC.: Great Barrington, MA. Primary source for Sproutman Steve Meyerowitz's sprouting supplies of all sorts, including a wide variety of seeds, sprouting baskets, sprouting bags, and *"Sprout Houses"* (mini-greenhouses for growing sprouts). Also, anyone who wants to optimize the possibilities for sprouting success must have Steve's book, *Sprouts the Miracle Food*, also available from The Sprout House, Inc. and at many health food stores. 1-800-SPROUTS. E-mail, sprout@sproutman.com   (H, M).

SPROUTING SUPPLIES and INSTRUCTION: A brand of sprouting seed available at most health food stores is Handy Pantry. Health food stores will often carry bulk sprouting seed for the most common sprouts, such as alfalfa and sunflower seed. Two books with detailed sprouting instructions are *Junk Food to Real Food*, by Carol Nostrand, and *Sprouts the Miracle Food* by Steve Meyerowitz. (See Recommended Bibliography. Also see SPROUT HOUSE, INC.)

SUPER-FOODS: Super-foods are food supplements made entirely from whole foods, which have a concentration of lively food-source nutrients. This category also includes everything in the GREEN-FOODS listing above. However, super-foods is a broader category than green-foods and as far as I am concerned, they are both important for health-conscious consumers to know about. Super-foods can keep you going through environmental pollution, job stress, traveling, and missed meals. They are tops for health maintenance and many of them are enjoyed by children. I use super-foods in place of synthetic vitamins for children because they are more fully assimilated and naturally used by the body without overwhelming it, as synthetic vitamins often do.

Super-foods are perfect for use during illness and recovery when potent, easy-to-assimilate nutrition is especially needed. If you think that you need extra "fuel" for your particular lifestyle, beyond what you get from a healthy diet high in the *10 Essential Foods*, one of these supplements may be for you. If you are traveling under stressfull circumstances, or where nutritious food may be scarce, all the more reason to try a couple of these super-foods and find out ahead of time which ones work the best for you. For myself, I find the *Klamath Blue Green Algae* (see GREEN-FOODS), a good ionic trace mineral product (see MINERALS), and the *Phyt-Aloe* or *Phyto-Bears* (see REJENITEC), together or separately, do a great job of super-fueling my activities and health. But, then again, I don't see how I would do without my *Papaya John's Energy Bars* on ocassion either! Look under the following headings (also see MAIL ORDER):

- BEE POLLEN
- **REJENITEC
- GARLIC
- GREEN-FOODS
- **PAPAYA JOHN'S ENERGY BARS*
  (see Snacks Appendix C)

SUPPLEMENTS: (see MAIL ORDER)

SWEETENERS: (see HONEY and MOLASSES)

TRACE MINERALS (ionic): (see MINERALS)

UMEBOSHI PLUM PASTE: (see EDEN FOODS)

VEGETABLE JUICERS: (see APPLIANCES)

VINEGAR: To get the full, famous, healing, health-enlivining results of vinegar, it must be unpasteurized. Use unpasteurized apple cider vinegar for salad dressings or any vinegar use. When you use the artificially aged, pasteurized vinegars as the major type of vinegar in food preparation, these add to the unhealthy acidity associated with many degenerative diseases such as arthritis. One detailed resource on the healing powers of "real" vinegar is the book, *Apple Cider Vinegar Health System,* by Paul and Patricia Bragg (both N.D. and Ph.D.). There are several good brands of unpasteurized apple vinegars such as Mantova, Bragg, and Hains, as well as this intriguing book, at health food stores. Or, to mail-order the Bragg's book, or their fantastic, unpasteurized, apple cider vinegar, call 1-800-446-1990. (G, H).

VITAMINS: (see MAIL ORDER)

WAKANUGA OF AMERICA: (see GARLIC)

WATER FILTERS:
PRES-2-PURE and *PUMP-N-PURE* from Global Water Tech. In the words of one water researcher and admirer of this product. "The units are the only ones proven to truly purify water by analytical studies performed by both commercial and government laboratories, including the State of California. Completely new technology. Invented by the man who introduced commercial reverse osmosis in 1971. These units are far superior and much less expensive than reverse osmosis." This new technology should be available in January of 1997. Contact Amvi Science Products, P.O. Box 1101, Tacoma, WA 98401. (206) 922-9113.
TAP DANCE water filtration systems from Natural Water Systems, Boulder, CO. In case you want something that does a decent job of filtering water while being within most people's budgets, check out these *Tap Dance* filters. Call 1-800-272-0982.
MICROWATER® SYSTEM distributed by Health Watchers System®, Scottsdale, AZ. This system is Japanese preventive-medicine technology, being made available in the United States. According to the literature, it not only filters water but also applies a patented electrolysis process to tap water, turning the water into a potent healing agent used in maintaining good health and strong immunity, as well for the treatment of illness including, but not limited to, poor digestion, chronic diarrhea, excess gastric acid, and skin disease. The pH of microwater® can be adjusted up or down for various healing purposes. Microwater® is

one of the most powerful antioxidants known. It is definitely worth investigating this further. Call Health Watchers at 1-800-321-6917. (M).

WHEAT GRASS AND BARLEY GRASS: (see GREEN-FOODS)

WHOLE GRAINS: (see BROWN RICE)

APPENDIX C

10 ESSENTIAL SNACKS

When I use the word "snacks" I am not suggesting the health-negative, habitual (perhaps addictive?) use of junky foods. Rather, I am advocating the strategic and intentional use of specific health-positive foods in quantities from "a few bites of something" to "light meals." These types of snacks are *strategic* because they can be used at crucial times during the day—like when your energy is flagging and additional nutrients and "body fuel" are needed to complete the task at hand, or when you don't want to be bogged down with a whole meal but you don't want to skip it altogether, either. These examples represent a far different mood than the one of randomly eating health-negative junk foods (or even their health-food equivalents) as a type of comfort during times of stress. On the other hand, these *10 Essential Snacks* are healthy ways to fuel yourself through stressful times when used properly. This is where the word *intentional* comes in. In the system of snacking I suggest, you will be strategically and intentionally using potent foods for health whenever you need them—nothing unconscious, health-negative, or addictive about it!

When I am traveling, or working on a deadline and skipping mealtimes, or living through an extremely hot summer day when I have little appetite, I depend on these snacks to give me the super-fuel I need while requiring the least digestive attention. This way, I stay energized and well-nourished, not over-fed and sluggish. Also, these *10 Essential Snacks* are useful for anyone intrigued by the idea of Conscious Undereating, which I write about in Guideline 10 of chapter 2.

For educating, or re-educating yourself and your children in the use of foods for health-positive snacks, there is no better, more health-promoting, or more painless place to start than with the following list:

1. CARROT JUICE (and other vegetable juices): Always try to drink your juice directly after it is made. This means that you are probably making it yourself with one of the handy appliances listed in Guideline 6 of chapter 2, or watching it being made for you at a juice bar. Second choice is bottled "fresh" vegetable juice. These always say they were "made fresh today," but don't you ever wonder if they really were? I do.

Try to get organic juice when you can. If you make your own carrot juice from non-organic carrots, remember to detoxify them as described in chapter 2. You will be very pleased with the results you get from using carrot juice as a snack food—steady energy, low calories, easy digestibility with no sluggishness afterwards and concentrated nutrition. Many adults are surprised to learn that their children love carrot juice. Younger children often like it diluted to varying degrees. Babies like it in their bottles, but be sure to strain it and dilute it half and half with pure water for them.

2. ESSENE BREAD (sweet, thick and sticky, sprouted-grain bread): Sometimes called *Manna Bread*, my favorite brand is Nature's Path *Manna Bread* and my favorite "flavor" (there are several) is the Sprouted Rye with carrot and raisin. Essene bread is made of sprouted whole grains prepared at low heat without preservatives, yeast, added sugars etc. It will be found in the frozen foods section at health food stores. Eat a hunk of this scrumptious, heavy yet cake-like bread, plain or with Seed Spread (#9 see below), fruit spread (fruit preserves made solely from fruit), butter, honey, or even mustard! See the Condiments list as well as Jams and Jellies in Supplies Appendix B, for more ideas of what can go with this bread. Also see more about Essene Sprouted Bread in the SHOPPING SKILLS and the KIDS LOVE THIS sections of the Sprout chapter.

3. FRUIT SMOOTHIES: These refreshing drinks are familiar to many, from the youngest to the oldest fruit enthusiasts. Smoothies make a perfect snack or light meal. You must have a blender, a Vita Mix machine (see Appendix B), or a food processor to perform the miracle from whole fruit to Fruit Smoothie. I suppose one could also grind and mash the fruit manually but the word "smoothie" would then have to be more loosely interpreted. The basic idea here is to gather a combination of fresh and/or frozen fruits into the food gadget/machine of choice and blend them together until smooth. The more frozen fruits you have in the mixture, the more of a thicker, sherbet-like frozen dessert texture you end up with. You can also get a thick and cool fruit drink by using ice cubes instead of frozen fruit and then the drink is less fruit-concentrated.

Many people mix all sorts of nuts and seeds and protein powders along with their fruit mixture but I would not recommend this. For ease of digestion and best absorption of nutrients, it is best to eat fruit alone and not mixed with other types of foods which, like the proteins in nuts, seeds and protein powders, are processed in the body far differently than the fruits. Indeed proteins and fruits, for example, often have conflicting sets of digestive processes (proteins: long and slow; fruits: short and fast) that need to take place to optimally utilize the nutrients in each, even if no digestive inconveniences become apparent. Exceptions to this are banana, or high-digestive-enzyme fruits such as Figs, papaya, pineapple or mango. If you are going to mix proteins into a Fruit Smoothie, it is a good idea to use one of these high-digestive-enzyme fruits either whole, as part of the mix, or in the juice used as the base liquid for the smoothie.

Although most people feel energized and wonderful from this Fruit Smoothie snack, if you feel a little "off" not long after a smoothie, it could be the particular mixture of ingredients that is getting to you. On the other hand, you might investigate whether or not you are simply getting too much fruit sugar for your metabolism. Perhaps you needed a different type of snack in that moment, such as Essene Bread, Popcorn, Yogurt, or Carrot or other vegetable juice. It pays off in health dividends to figure these things out!

4.   FROZEN JUICE POPS: These are made by simply freezing a favorite juice (some people even freeze left-over fruit smoothie), but there are definitely tricks that one must learn. First of all, read the juice labels. Did you know that even in the frozen juice concentrates with luscious sounding names you may only be getting 30% juice? You want 100% juice with no sugar added, so you've got to read the label. Buy a plastic "popsicle" mold with the accompanying hand-holders to freeze the juice pops in, or fill small paper cups or something like that, with the juice and use plastic spoons (or whatever) for the handles. If you use this paper cup method, don't make the mistake of making the juice pops too large because then you can't properly get one into your mouth, so it is not as much fun to eat. Needless to say, children love these juice pop snacks. Even our refrigerator repair man loves these! When he came to fix the refrigerator he got all hot and sweaty (after all we live in Arizona and it was a hot summer day, even indoors). There on the counter sat the juice pops, melting because we had to remove them from the freezer for the repairs. He spied the grape ones and remarked, "Those look refreshing." Whereupon we offered him one. He loved it!

5. PAPAYA JOHN'S ENERGY BARS: There is actually a man named John who lives in Hawaii, where he makes these great energy/snack/health bars. They weigh 1/4 pound each and are about 7 inches long by 3 1/2 inches wide. These bars come in several flavors, and all ingredients are organic! The main ingredient is papaya with varying amounts of one or more of the following: Figs, apples, bee pollen, spirulina, apricots, lemon juice, whey, Almonds, dates, sesame, fresh ginger and more. So far, the flavors are Papaya-almond, Papaya-macadamia nut, Papaya-sesame, Papaya-fruit, Papaya-ginger and Papaya-protein nutrition (it has spirulina, a type of nutritionally-potent algae in it). My personal favorites are the Papaya-ginger and the Papaya-protein nutrition bars. As a snack, you only need to eat a bite or two at a time to get adequate fuel for energy. I suppose an active person could down a whole bar at one sitting, but let me tell you, I am an active person and one bar lasts me several days! The papaya and Figs are such a help to aid digestion that it also works well to take a bite or two of a *Papaya John's Energy Bar* before or after a meal (the papaya-ginger is especially good in this regard). Fantastic! The only way to get them, however, unless you live near Papaya John, is by mail order. Take a tip from me and order at least six at a time. This saves you postage and later on it saves you from running out and having to wait for more. Papaya John also makes the most incredible thin, marmalade-type spread called *Papaya Concentrate.* Buy a quart of this ambrosia for your snacks. WOW! As of this writing (Spring 1997), his prices are $6.25 for one bar and the price goes down if you buy two or more. The *Papaya Concentrate* is $20 per quart, and less for a gallon. Shipping is $6.50 for every 4 lbs. Write, call, or FAX to him. Papaya John, P.O. Box 441, Paia, Maui, HI 96779. (808) 579-9608, FAX (808) 573-0128. Delivery is very fast.

6. PICKLES: Cucumber Pickles and other pickled, marinated or fermented raw vegetables, such as sauerkraut or an ad-lib mixture of one's own, make great snacks. However, you should be careful about the quality of what you buy because you can get a lot of junky stuff passed off as pickles, sauerkraut, or marinated vegetables at grocery stores. At the health food store you can buy real pickles, etc., without food colorings, preservatives, or "synthetic" vinegars and with much less, or no, salt; and they may be even organic! (Also see the Pickles, Ginger Pickles and Sea Pickles listings in Supplies Appendix B.)

7. POPCORN: This snack is so versatile that it can be taken anywhere. I took popcorn kernels to India once and had some village friends cook it. They heated up some fine sand in an iron-looking skillet and when the sand got hot, they threw in the popcorn and let it pop out of the uncovered pan onto the hard-packed clay ground, which had been carefully swept for the event. Here it was picked up by the children and myself, a few kernels at a time. The faster it popped, the faster we scurried after it to prevent the birds or other foragers from getting there first.

Popcorn! You can sauce it a hundred different ways, use it as a breakfast cereal, stick it together in balls with a cooked honey syrup, or stuff yourself with it (like I do, along with the green drink described in the TASOLE in the Spinach chapter) for a light dinner meal once in awhile. In my book *10 Essential Herbs*, I suggest eating Garlic Popcorn, using a sauce of fresh garlic and olive oil, as a delicious concoction for pleasure or for medicinal purposes. See the creative, good-tasting popcorn seasoning recipe in the Dulse chapter.

8. RICE CAKES: These 1/2-inch-thick puffed-rice crackers are found at most grocery stores and at absolutely every self-respecting health food store. (They measure 5 inches in diameter.) Having minimal calories and a mild neutral taste, rice cakes make a crunchy base for jams, jellies (fruit preserves) and seed spread/nut butters (see the KIDS LOVE THIS idea in the Almond chapter and the Seed Balls recipe below). Also, I suggest using honey and/or butter on rice cakes, or whatever you would normally put on a crackers. Be sure to buy whole grain Brown Rice cakes and not the ones made with milled white rice (which are lacking in the whole grain nutrients and possibly include some similar things to the nutrient-deficient, additive-laden, bleached white flour breads).

9. **SEED BALLS and SPREADS:** This idea is written up in the Almond chapter and I repeat it here. A variety of seeds and nuts could be used but the basic idea is the same. Eat these "balls and spreads" alone, or on crackers, rice cakes, or bread. They make a good snack combination with Carrot juice.

In a blender, food processor, or coffee bean/nut grinder, grind fresh, raw Almonds to a powder. As an alternative you may want to grind a variety of seeds such as an Almond, sunflower seed, pumpkin seed, sesame seed combination. Grind enough to get one cup of powdered Almonds, or whatever mix you like. A good trick is to lightly dry roast the sesame seeds (using no oil) in a hot skillet before grinding them; but do not roast the other nuts or seeds. (Anytime you heat raw nuts and seeds you are damaging their oils and thus their digestibility. With sesame, a very light roasting does little damage.) This dry-roasted sesame gives a particularly "nutty" flavor.

Grind until you have the texture that suits you. To each cup of this nut/seed powder, add two tablespoons of a healthy oil such as cold pressed *Barlean's Organic Flaxseed Oil*, sesame, sunflower, olive oil or Almond oil and two tablespoons of pure water. Continue to add water until you get a consistency somewhat like sticky clay, if you are making seed balls; or, add water until a looser consistency is achieved if you intend to spread it, or looser still if you intend to use it as a vegetable dip. You can add a dollop of honey to this mixture if you like. As a spread it is easily adaptable for use in sandwiches, appetizers, or stuffed vegetable finger-foods such as stuffed celery stalks, carrot sticks, etc.

When making seed balls, mold the thicker, sticky mixture into a ball the size of your liking. If desired, for a sweeter result roll these balls in a mixture of shredded coconut and/or roasted carob powder (a light brown, sweet and tasty powder of the carob bean available at health food stores). For a saltier result, roll these balls in powdered Dulse or the *Sea Seasonings* mentioned under Maine Coast Sea Vegetables in Supplies Appendix B.

Be certain to keep these fresh seed mixtures refrigerated; they will preserve quite well for a week or two. They can also be frozen for longer storage. Serve these nut-seed balls as a high-protein, high calorie, high-energy snack for active people.

10. YOGURT—LIVE CULTURE: The type of yogurt I am suggesting for a snack is the "real" kind. It will still have significant amounts of living yogurt cultures/bacteria. (Live cultures/bacteria must be added back to the milk *after* the pasteurizing process. Some manufacturers pasteurize their yogurt *after* they culture it. This effectively "kills" it. Some add back the living culture, but some do not. Some companies pasteurize their milk and then culture it, which makes more sense to me. In both cases they can call it yogurt.)

If it is *live culture* yogurt, you would be able to use some of it as a starter to make more yogurt, if you felt like it. If it is the other kind, what I call the "pretend kind," you could probably glue envelopes shut with it when it got old. You can check out whether yogurt is guaranteed to have living healthy bacteria (yogurt cultures) by reading the label. You'll be getting a synthetic variety of yogurt unless you check this out.

Have you ever noticed all the choices of yogurt at stores? When you read the labels you see that there is a wide variety of additives that some manufacturers put into their products. Examples of these additives are gelatin, tapioca, sugars, colorings, flavorings, oils and even preservatives.

If you get living-culture yogurt, with as few additives as possible, you'll have a satisfying snack with the health-positive parts of yogurt still present. My favorite mix is plain yogurt with my own honey and dash of nutmeg added.

INDEX

For each of the *Ten Essential Foods*, see also Alternatives; Functional Components; Healthy Additions; Kids Love This; Survival Choices; Travelers Tips.

ADDITIONAL TITLES OF INTEREST FROM HOHM PRESS

YOUR BODY CAN TALK: How to Listen to What Your Body Knows and Needs Through Simple Muscle Testing
by Susan L. Levy, D.C. and Carol Lehr, M.A.

Imagine having a diagnostic tool so sensitive that it could immediately tell you: • exactly how much protein...or fat...Your Body needs...• precisely which vitamins and minerals are needed in Your Diet...• what particular factors in the environment are depleting Your Vital Energy...• what hidden allergies you may have • which organs in your body are weakened due to over-stress • or anything else related to your health and well-being. You Already Have This Tool...at your own fingertips. Dr. Levy and Carol Lehr present clear instructions in *simple muscle testing*, together with over 25 simple tests for how to use it for specific problems or disease conditions. Special chapters deal with health problems specific to women (especially PMS and Menopause) and problems specific to men (like stress, heart disease, and prostate difficulties). Contains over 30 diagrams, plus a complete Index and Resource Guide.

Paper, 350 pages, $19.95, ISBN: 0-934252-68-8

• • •

NATURAL HEALING WITH HERBS
by Humbart "Smokey" Santillo, N.D.
Foreword by Robert S. Mendelsohn, M.D.

Dr. Santillo's first book, and Hohm Press' long-standing bestseller, is a classic handbook on herbal and naturopathic treatment. Acclaimed as the most comprehensive work of its kind, *Natural Healing With Herbs* details (in layperson's terms) the properties and uses of 120 of the most common herbs and lists comprehensive therapies for more than 140 common ailments. All in alphabetical order for quick reference.
Includes special sections on: • Diagnosis • How to make herbal remedies • The nature of health and disease • Diet and detoxification • Homeopathy... and more

Over 150,000 copies in print.
Paper, 408 pages, $16.95, ISBN: 0-934252-08-4

TO ORDER, PLEASE SEE ACCOMPANYING ORDER FORM.

ADDITIONAL TITLES OF INTEREST FROM HOHM PRESS

FOOD ENZYMES: THE MISSING LINK TO RADIANT HEALTH
by Humbart "Smokey" Santillo, N.D.

Immune system health is a subject of concern for everyone today. This book explains how the body's immune system, as well as every other human metabolic function, requires enzymes in order to work properly. Food enzyme supplementation is more essential today than ever before, since stress, unhealthy food, and environmental pollutants readily deplete them from the body. Humbart Santillo's breakthrough book presents the most current research in this field, and encourages simple, straightforward steps for how to make enzyme supplementation a natural addition to a nutrition-conscious lifestyle.

Special sections on: • Longevity and disease • The value of raw food and juicing • Detoxification • Prevention of allergies and candida • Sports and nutrition

Over 200,000 copies in print.
Paper, 108 pages, U.S. $7.95, ISBN: 0-934252-40-8 (English)

Now available in Spanish language version.
Paper, 108 pages, U.S. $6.95, ISBN: 0-934252-49-1 (Spanish)

■ Audio version of Food Enzymes
2 cassette tapes, 150 minutes, U.S. $17.95, ISBN: 0-934252-29-7

• • •

INTUITIVE EATING: EveryBody's Guide to Vibrant Health and Lifelong Vitality Through Food
by Humbart "Smokey" Santillo, N.D.

The natural voice of the body has been drowned out by the shouts of addictions, over-consumption, and devitalized and preserved foods. Millions battle the scale daily, experimenting with diets and nutritional programs, only to find their victories short-lived at best, confusing and demoralizing at worst. *Intuitive Eating* offers an alternative—a tested method for: • strengthening the immune system • natural weight loss • increasing energy • making the transition from a degenerative diet to a regenerative diet • slowing the aging process.

Paper, 450 pages, $16.95, ISBN: 0-934252-27-0

TO ORDER, PLEASE SEE ACCOMPANYING ORDER FORM.

ADDITIONAL TITLES OF INTEREST FROM HOHM PRESS

10 ESSENTIAL HERBS, REVISED EDITION
by Lalitha Thomas

Peppermint. . .Garlic. . .Ginger. . .Cayenne. . .Clove. . . and 5 other everyday herbs win the author's vote as the "Top 10" most versatile and effective herbal applications for hundreds of health and beauty needs. *Ten Essential Herbs* offers fascinating stories and easy, step-by-step direction for both beginners and seasoned herbalists. Learn how to use cayenne for headaches, how to make a facial scrub with ginger, how to calm motion sickness and other stomach distress with peppermint, how to make slippery-elm cough drops for sore-throat relief. Special sections in each chapter explain the application of these herbs with children and pets too.
Over 25,000 copies in print.

Paper, 395 pages, $16.95, ISBN: 0-934252-48-3

• • •

DHEA: THE ULTIMATE REJUVENATING HORMONE
by Hasnain Walji, Ph.D.

A sane and balanced approach to the use of this age-slowing hormone, DHEA, which is fast being acknowledged as a new "wonder substance." Many studies indicate DHEA's positive usage for athletes and others concerned with losing weight without reducing caloric intake (DHEA blocks a fat-producing enzyme), as an aid to both short and long-term memory loss, and in such conditions as diabetes, cancer, Chronic Fatigue Syndrome, heart disease and immune system deficiencies. Contains a comprehensive but user-friendly review of research and relevant nutritional information.

Paper, 95 pages, $9. 95, ISBN: 0-934252-70-X

TO ORDER, PLEASE SEE ACCOMPANYING ORDER FORM.

ADDITIONAL TITLES OF INTEREST FROM HOHM PRESS

ARE YOU GETTING IT 5 TIMES A DAY?
Fruits and Vegetables
by Sydney H. Crackower, M.D., Barry A. Bohn, M.D. and
Rodney Langlinais, Reg. Pharmacist

The evidence is irrefutable. Research from around the world, and from
the American Cancer Society and the National Cancer Institute in the
U.S. agree ... 5 servings of nature's disease fighters—raw fruits and
vegetables—would markedly reduce cancer...stroke...and heart disease,
the leading killers of our times. Fresh fruits and vegetables, as well as an
intelligently pursued regimen of antioxidants, live enzymes and high fiber
are the nutritional basics of good health. This concise and straightforward
book will give you all the background research and practical steps you
need to start getting it today!

Paper, 78 pages, $ 6.95, ISBN: 0-934252-35-1

• • •

■ *HERBS, NUTRITION AND HEALING ;* AUDIO CASSETTE SERIES
by Dr. Humbart "Smokey" Santillo, N.D.

Santillo's most comprehensive seminar series. Topics covered in-depth
include: • the history of herbology • specific preparation of herbs for
tinctures, salves, concentrates, etc. • herbal dosages in both acute and
chronic illnesses • use of cleansing and transition diets • treating colds
and flu... and more.

4 cassettes, 330 minutes, $40.00, ISBN: 0-934252-22-X

• • •

■ *NATURE HEALS FROM WITHIN;* AUDIO CASSETTE SERIES
by Dr. Humbart "Smokey" Santillo, N.D.

How to take the next step in improving your life and health through
nutrition. Topics include: • The innate wisdom of the body. • The essential
role of elimination and detoxification • Improving digestion • How
"transition dieting" will take off the weight—for good! • The role of
heredity, diet, and prevention in health • How to overcome tiredness,
improve your immune system and live longer...and happier.

1 cassette, $8.95, ISBN: 0-934252-66-1

TO ORDER, PLEASE SEE ACCOMPANYING ORDER FORM.

ADDITIONAL TITLES OF INTEREST FROM HOHM PRESS

■ *LIVE SEMINAR ON FOOD ENZYMES*; AUDIO CASSETTE SERIES
by Dr. Humbart "Smokey" Santillo, N.D.

An in-depth discussion of the properties of food enzymes, describing their valuable use to maintain vitality, immunity, health and longevity. A must for anyone interested in optimal health. Complements all the information in the book.

1 cassette, $8.95, ISBN: 0-934252-29-7

• • •

■ *FRUITS AND VEGETABLES—The Basis of Health*; AUDIO CASSETTE SERIES
by Dr. Humbart "Smokey" Santillo, N.D.

Juicing of fruits and vegetables is one of the fastest and most efficient ways to supply the body with the raw food nutrients and enzymes needed to maintain optimal health. Explains the essential difference between a live food diet, which heals the body, and degenerative foods, which weaken the immune system and cause disease. Recipes included.

1 cassette, $8.95, ISBN: 0-934252-65-3

• • •

■ *WEIGHT-LOSS SEMINAR*; AUDIO CASSETTE SERIES
by Dr. Humbart "Smokey" Santillo, N.D.

"The healthiest people in the world know the secret of weight loss," says Santillo in this candid, practical, and information-based seminar. "If your body is getting what it needs, the appetite automatically turns off!" The reason for overweight is that we are starving ourselves to death, based on the improper balance of nutrients from our current food sources. This seminar explains the worthlessness of most dietary regimens and explodes many common myths about weight gain. Santillo stresses: • The essential distinction between "good" fats and "bad" fats • The necessity for protein and how to use it efficiently • How to get our primary vitamins and minerals from food • How to ease into becoming an "intuitive eater" so that the body is always getting what it knows it needs.

1 cassette, $8.95, ISBN: 0-934252-75-0

TO ORDER, PLEASE SEE ACCOMPANYING ORDER FORM.

ADDITIONAL TITLES OF INTEREST FROM HOHM PRESS

10 ESSENTIAL FOODS
by Lalitha Thomas

Lalitha has done for food what she did with such wit and wisdom for herbs in her best-selling *10 Essential Herbs*. This new book presents 10 ordinary, but *essential* and great-tasting foods that can: • Strengthen a weakened immune system • Rebalance brain chemistry • Fight cancer and other degenerative diseases • Help you lose weight, simply and naturally.

Carrots, broccoli, almonds, grapefruit and six other miracle foods will enhance your health when used regularly and wisely. Lalitha gives in-depth nutritional information plus flamboyant and good-humored stories about these foods, based on her years of health and nutrition counseling. Each chapter contains easy and delicious recipes, tips for feeding kids and helpful hints for managing your food dollar. A bonus section supports the use of 10 Essential Snacks.

"This book's focus is squarely on target: fruits, vegetables and whole grains—everything comes in the right natural proportions."—Charles Attwood, M.D., F.A.A.P.; author, *Dr. Attwoods Low-Fat Prescription for Kids* (Viking).

Paper, 300 pages, $16.95, ISBN: 0-934252-74-2

• • •

THE MELATONIN AND AGING SOURCEBOOK
by Dr. Roman Rozencwaig, M.D. and Dr. Hasnain Walji, Ph.D.

"This is the most comprehensive reference on melatonin, yet published. It is an indispensable tool for those scientists, researchers, and physicians engaged in anti-aging therapeutics." —Dr. Ronald Klatz, President, American Academy of Anti-aging Medicing

This book covers the latest research on the pineal...control of aging, melatonin and sleep, melatonin and immunity, melatonin's role in cancer treatment, antioxidant qualities of melatonin, dosages, counter indications, quality control, and use with other drugs, melatonin application to heart disease, Alzheimer's, diabetes, stress, major depression, seasonal affective disorders, AIDS, SIDS, cataracts, autism...and many other conditions.

Cloth, 220 pages, $79.95, ISBN: 0-934252-73-4

TO ORDER, PLEASE SEE ACCOMPANYING ORDER FORM.

RETAIL ORDER FORM FOR HOHM PRESS HEALTH BOOKS

Name_____ Phone (   ) _____

Street Address or P.O. Box _____

City _____State _____ Zip Code _____

	QTY	TITLE	ITEM PRICE	TOTAL PRICE
1		10 ESSENTIAL FOODS	$16.95	
2		10 ESSENTIAL HERBS	$16.95	
3		ARE YOU GETTING IT 5 TIMES A DAY?	$6.95	
4		DHEA: The Ultimate Rejuvenating Hormone	$9.95	
5		FOOD ENZYMES/ENGLISH	$7.95	
6		FOOD ENZYMES/SPANISH	$6.95	
7		FOOD ENZYMES BOOK/AUDIO	$17.95	
8		FRUITS & VEGETABLES/AUDIO	$8.95	
9		HERBS, NUTRITION AND HEALING/AUDIO	$40.00	
10		INTUITIVE EATING	$16.95	
11		LIVE SEMINAR ON FOOD ENZYMES/AUDIO	$8.95	
12		THE MELATONIN AND AGING SOURCEBOOK	$79.95	
13		NATURAL HEALING WITH HERBS	$16.95	
14		NATURE HEALS FROM WITHIN/AUDIO	$8.95	
15		WEIGHT LOSS SEMINAR/AUDIO	$8.95	
16		YOUR BODY CAN TALK: How to Listen...	$19.95	

SURFACE SHIPPING CHARGES
1st book $4.00
Each additional item $1.00

SUBTOTAL:
SHIPPING: (see below)
TOTAL:

SHIP MY ORDER

☐ Surface U.S. Mail—Priority   ☐ UPS (Mail + $2.00)
☐ 2nd-Day Air (Mail + $5.00)   ☐ Next-Day Air (Mail + $15.00)

METHOD OF PAYMENT:

☐ Check or M.O.   Payable to Hohm Press, P.O. Box 2501, Prescott, AZ 86302
☐ Call 1-800-381-2700 to place your credit card order
☐ Or call 1-520-717-1779 to fax your credit card order
☐ Information for Visa/MasterCard order only:

Card #_____-_____-_____-_____   Expiration Date _____

ORDER NOW! Call 1-800-381-2700 or fax your order to 1-520-717-1779.
(Remember to include your credit card information.)